Dialectical Behavior Therapy for Sex Offenders

This treatment guide allows clinicians to effectively integrate dialectical behavior therapy (DBT) as a psychological treatment for men who have committed sexually motivated offenses.

It provides clinicians with the most current, evidence-based research about sex offenders' risks and treatment needs, and draws upon the therapeutic techniques of DBT and cognitive behavioral therapy. The guide is divided into five parts that provide practical, evidence-based skills for clients to apply to their lives to reduce the likelihood of recidivism. It explores numerous skill sets that target all major areas of dysregulation commonly seen among men who have committed sexual offences. Worksheets, images, group discussion ideas, and roleplay scenarios are used throughout to help clients practice their skills within the group setting and on their own.

This guide is essential for all mental health professionals who work with men who have committed sexual crimes.

Dr Abigail Kolb, Ph.D., is an associate professor of criminology at the University of West Georgia. Her research has primarily focused on gender and offending. She is also a licensed social worker and has worked in forensic mental health for over a decade, focusing on the treatment of sexual offenders. As a trained DBT practitioner, she hopes to help other clinicians implement this treatment modality for sex offenders.

Dialectical Behavior Therapy for Sex Offenders

A Treatment Guide

ABIGAIL KOLB

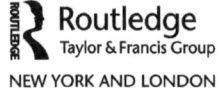
Routledge
Taylor & Francis Group

NEW YORK AND LONDON

Designed cover image: Khanchit Khirisutchalual © Getty Images

First published 2024
by Routledge
605 Third Avenue, New York, NY 10158

and by Routledge
4 Park Square, Milton Park, Abingdon, Oxon, OX14 4RN

Routledge is an imprint of the Taylor & Francis Group, an informa business

Library of Congress Cataloging-in-Publication Data
Names: Kolb, Abigail, author.
Title: Dialectical behavior therapy for sex offenders : a treatment guide / Abigail Kolb.
Description: New York, NY : Routledge, 2024. | Includes bibliographical references and index. |
Identifiers: LCCN 2023038794 (print) | LCCN 2023038795 (ebook) | ISBN 9781032586960 (pbk) | ISBN 9781032586977 (hbk) | ISBN 9781003451099 (ebk)
Subjects: LCSH: Sex offenders—Rehabilitation. | Dialectical behavior therapy. | Sex offenders—Mental health. | Sex offenders—Mental health services.
Classification: LCC RC560.S47 K65 2024 (print) | LCC RC560.S47 (ebook) | DDC 364.15/3–dc23/eng/20231103
LC record available at https://lccn.loc.gov/2023038794
LC ebook record available at https://lccn.loc.gov/2023038795

ISBN: 978-1-032-58697-7 (hbk)
ISBN: 978-1-032-58696-0 (pbk)
ISBN: 978-1-003-45109-9 (ebk)

DOI: 10.4324/9781003451099

Typeset in Dante and Avenir
by codeMantra

Access the Support Material: www.routledge.com/9781032586960

I dedicate this to my michpocha: Andreas, Mom, Pop, Leah, Stuart, and "the kids."

Contents

Acknowledgments

This work was a labor of love that kept me busy when I was not teaching or seeing clients. I first learned about dialectical behavior therapy (DBT) in graduate school, while taking a class with the professor whom I will forever consider my mentor, Dr. Andre Ivanoff. Since then, I have practiced DBT in various clinical settings, including with men who have committed sexually motivated offenses. This work would not have been possible without the collaboration, support, and patience of my other mentor, Dr. Henry Schmidt III. Thank you, Henry, for all of your time and for making this a reality by always being there to "talk things through" and share your insights.

I wish to extend my deepest gratitude to Dr. Joseph Sakdalan for reviewing my work and providing such helpful feedback. I know how busy you are, and in taking the time to assist me you went above and beyond. Thank you for your willingness to answer my questions and share your insights and experience. Your reconceptualization of wise mind and the hierarchy of treatment targets is nothing short of brilliant and has contributed greatly to this field.

Furthermore, thanks to the amazing Lyne Piche and Anton Schweighoffer for your support and feedback on this project. Thanks to colleagues Kevin Baldwin and Rex Tuten. To my colleagues and friends Ericka Wentz, Gavin Lee, Lynn Pazzani, Tiffany Parsons, Felicia Johnson, Jennifer Martwick, and Kaley Zimmerman, thank you for the fun and laughs throughout, and for bearing with me. I will resume answering my phone and text messages.

Thank you to Sarah Rae, Pragati Sharma, Jana Craddock, and all of the wonderful people at Routledge for your help and support.

My mother, Jill; father, William; sister, Leah; and brother-in-law, Stuart; my husband, Andreas—the incredibly patient man who supports and puts up with me; and finally, our babies—Tiger, Dolly, Manny, and Chloe.

More generally, this would not have happened without the extensive research and work conducted by numerous experts in DBT and sex offender treatment.

Many years ago, Dr. Erika Horwitz, cultivated my understanding and practice of mindful living and interdependence. It has been a long, exhilarating journey, with ups and downs—as is life. However, nothing is possible without others. I am truly grateful to everyone mentioned here and many others who have been instrumental in helping me shape my career and do the work I love. I thank you from the bottom of my heart.

Introduction

Current cognitive behavioral interventions have been the gold standard when it comes to treating individuals convicted of sex crimes and reducing sexual recidivism. However, dialectical behavior therapy (DBT) has gained tremendous support as a third-wave cognitive behavioral treatment over the last three decades, and has demonstrated clinical efficacy to treat a variety of psychosocial conditions. DBT is unique in that it uses a dialectical approach that combines components of both Eastern philosophy (mindfulness) and traditional cognitive behavioral therapy (CBT). Cognitive behavioral approaches, when combined with mindfulness, have demonstrated empirical validity for addressing a wide range of psychosocial dysfunction, including emotional dysregulation, poor sense of identity, impulsivity, and interpersonal problems.[1]

DBT is a unique therapeutic modality developed in 1993 by psychologist Marsha Linehan to treat individuals suffering from borderline personality disorder. Since then, this treatment has been adapted to treat numerous populations suffering from mental health problems and compulsive behaviors such as substance abuse disorders,[2] aggressive behaviors,[3] and post-traumatic stress disorders.[4] DBT has been adapted to address the treatment needs of forensic samples—such as impulsive, aggressive incarcerated men[5] stalking offenders,[6] forensic inpatient samples,[7] men with borderline and antisocial personality disorder,[8] and individuals with antisocial personality disorder[9]—to reduce anger, aggression, and poor impulse control, as well as increase self-soothing and cognitive restructuring.[10] Given the challenging and intensive nature of DBT, it is crucial that individuals have a clear understanding of what DBT entails and what their role in the treatment process will be.

DOI: 10.4324/9781003451099-1

While many sex offence-specific clinicians have reported using elements of DBT in their treatment groups, the field has lacked a dedicated treatment guide that maintains the integrity of Linehan's model and applies it to sex offence-specific treatment. While DBT was not created specifically for treatment of individuals who have committed sexually motivated offences, clinicians and scholars note that it could be a highly effective treatment model, because there is significant overlap in major areas of dysregulation—specifically, emotional dysregulation—between those who commit sexually motivated offences and other populations with mental health disorders and compulsive behaviors.[11] Further, despite its alignment with the extant literature on use of CBT with sexual offenders, and the use of elements of DBT in sex offender treatment,[12] no comprehensive DBT treatment guide has been created to assist clinicians, to the best of my knowledge. As such, this guide serves as a proposed adaptation for clinicians and researchers interested in applying DBT to work with sexual offenders in the mainstream population, including incarcerated men and men within a treatment program in a community setting.

Research has consistently demonstrated that the risks of reoffending for men who commit sexually motivated offences include the following areas of dysregulation: poor interpersonal skills/social network, poor emotional regulation, problematic sexual regulation, and challenges tolerating distressing situations.[13] DBT addresses each of these domains except sexual regulation skills—a crucial component of sex offender treatment.

Theoretical Underpinnings

Similar to other treatment models rooted in positive psychology, DBT emphasizes quality of life, and uses a strengths-based approach similar the Good Lives Model[14] to address various areas of dysregulation in an individual's life. Additionally, this treatment model acknowledges that clients engage in harmful behavior as a means of attaining socially desired goals, but not having adequate resources to do so.[15] As such, my rationale for using DBT with men who have committed sexually motived offences is sixfold.

First, DBT is unique in that it acknowledges that changing distorted cognitions alone does not necessarily address clients' struggles with their fundamental self-regulatory foundation and ineffective management of affective states. In other words, DBT addresses underlying principles, skills, and processes that support and enable effective self-regulation through validation in order to help the client work toward change and achieve a life more worth living.

Second, incorporating DBT's biosocial theory has demonstrated efficacy in explaining the origin/development of other personality disorders such as antisocial personality and psychopathy, which are frequently observed in forensic settings,[16, 17] and at higher rates among sexual offenders when compared to non-sexual offenders.[18] DBT's biosocial theory suggests that there exists an interplay between biological factors and environmental influences that contributes to the development of personality disorders, and future sexual offending. Specifically, research has demonstrated that growing up in an invalidating environment contributes to persistent emotional and sexual dysregulation.[19] Application of this theory has helped researchers and practitioners understand and explain etiological factors and mechanisms implicated in personality disorders, sexual offending, and other psychosocial dysfunctions.

Third, DBT maintains a dialectical approach which is rooted in the assumption that opposing forces or ideas can be synthesized through a process of dialog and acceptance. At the heart of dialectics is the assumption that the individual is part of and interacts with larger systems (e.g., the whole "self," family, friends, school, the criminal justice system); and thus that treatment providers must address the mutually constitutive role of the person and their environment—an idea Linehan terms "reciprocal determinism." According to Levins and Lewontin (1985),[20] "these are the properties of things we call dialectical: that one thing cannot exist without the other, that one acquires its properties in relation to the other, that the properties of both evolve as a consequence of their interpretation." Thus, a dialectical perspective means that individuals can have two seemingly opposite ideas at the same time and find a way to reconcile them.

The fourth distinct feature of this treatment is that DBT stresses the importance of mindfulness and acceptance of feelings as they are in the moment. By incorporating the mindfulness component of treatment, Linehan demonstrated that clients can learn to observe their thoughts, feelings, and sensations without judgment or avoidance; and that by doing so, they can become more aware of their emotions and develop skills to regulate them.

Fifth, DBT primarily targets emotional dysregulation and self-harm behaviors that interfere with one's ability to achieve a life worth living, or wise life,[21] or that interfere with treatment; and uses a wide range of strategies and skill sets to teach emotion regulation, interpersonal effectiveness, and distress tolerance. In this guide, I argue that attaining skills mastery in these various areas of dysregulation reduces the harmful thoughts and behaviors, or sexual dynamic risk factors,[22] that make it more likely an individual will reoffend.

Finally, research has shown that DBT adaptations for forensic (correctional and psychiatric) populations adhere to the risk-needs-responsivity (RNR) model, which is an empirically supported model for addressing criminality.[23] This model has consistently supported the need for clinicians to address an individual's risk level. Ideally, treatment is targeted toward individuals that pose the highest risk of reoffence. Since DBT was developed to address individuals at high risk of self-harm and other risky behaviors, this intensive therapeutic model is suitable for higher-risk offenders. The clinician must also continuously assess and identify the individual's criminogenic needs in order to tailor individually responsive treatment to reduce recidivism. Implementation of this model is a necessary component in the treatment of sexually motivated offenders. Thus, adaptation of DBT for criminal populations aligns with the RNR model and is arguably well suited to treat men who have committed sexually motivated offences.

This guide provides an adaptation of various components of DBT for work with sexually motivated offenders. First, I have simplified the language throughout the guide in order to align with typical reading and comprehension levels among correctional populations.[24] Second, I have included a discussion of how to address the dynamic and acute stable risk factors from a dialectical perspective. Finally, I have added a section that addresses sexual regulation skills, as there is a strong link between dysregulation in this area and sexual deviance. Additionally, the manual includes worksheets, psychoeducational information for therapists to present to clients, group discussion ideas, and roleplay scenarios to help clients practice their skills within the group setting.

Style

If you are using this treatment guide, you are likely a licensed clinician and are thus familiar with the various assessment tools; can assess and identify your clients' level of comprehension, risk level, and criminogenic needs; and can implement the necessary responsivity principles to address those needs. As we know, there is no "one size fits all" treatment for any population. Numerous skill sets are presented throughout this guide. While this may seem overwhelming to clinicians and/or clients, remember that—as always—one skill set may work well for one client, but not for another. Thus, it is the skills trainers' role to teach a variety of skill sets, so clients have options. Individual therapists are then encouraged to help clients determine which specific skill sets they can implement in their lives—something which provides flexibility in, and individualization of, the individual's treatment process.

This guide provides ideas about how to teach the material in a clear, straightforward manner; however, you are not expected or encouraged to read the dialog to clients word for word. Instead, you are encouraged to use your clinical judgment to consider a "what works" approach with your treatment group(s) and individual clients, and tailor the material accordingly.

Skills training can be a tedious and often repetitive task for clinicians and clients. You will notice similar patterns and trends throughout the manual. Repetition in skills training is crucial in order to help clients understand basic skills, continuously build upon them, and ensure the transferability of those skills in various contexts and situations.[25] Various concepts and skill sets are included in this manual to address clients' psychosocial and psychosexual challenges.

This treatment guide consists of five parts and 18 chapters. The chapters do not necessarily equate to one full session; rather, the skills trainers will decide which and how much material to teach in each session. Ideally, skills training groups will be completed in two or three-hour sessions once or twice per week, and one-hour individual sessions per week. The skills trainer's role is to teach the skills during group; while the individual therapist will address the treatment targets discussed in Chapter 1 and reinforce the client's daily use of the skills they learned in group. Depending on the time and resources provided at your facility/agency, clients are encouraged to repeat DBT training in cycles; however, you may choose which skills you prefer to teach based on the risk level of the group and individual with whom you are working. In addition to the skills training group, it is strongly recommended that clients attend individual therapy for at least one hour per week. Adherence to the RNR principles is essential to adequately address clients' criminogenic needs, while tailoring responsivity measures to the individual.[26] While there have been inconsistencies about preferred treatment length and intensity, [27] Correctional Service Canada (CSC) suggests that 24–60 hours is sufficient to reduce recidivism for lower-risk offenders. Furthermore, CSC recommends 160–200 contact hours for moderate-risk offenders, and 360–540 contact hours for high-risk offenders.[28] Considering that there are numerous skill sets presented here, and that clients tend to absorb material more with repetition, which affords them the opportunity to practice their skills, it would be ideal to provide the program back-to-back for higher-risk clients.

Overview

Part I: Summary

Chapter 1 provides clinicians with an overview of DBT, treatment targets, and therapy-interfering behaviors, and discusses the various components necessary to develop DBT programming at their facility, while maintaining the integrity of Linehan's modality. Chapter 2 introduces the individual therapist(s) concepts and materials during the initial individual treatment sessions, and how to familiarize clients with specific concepts that will be used throughout treatment. Clients will become oriented with the DBT skills model; address the importance of prosocial relationships; and consider long and short-term goals, and their readiness for changing behaviors that interfere with their goals for living a wise life. They will learn how to fill out a daily diary to keep track of skills practice, and how to critically analyze their behaviors using two types of functional analyses: behavior chain analysis and missing link analysis. In the following two chapters, clinicians will address group dynamics and ask clients to create a list of expectations to ensure group cohesiveness and safety. Clinicians will also explain various biological, psychological, and social factors that have been implicated in sexual offending to provide clients with a foundation for understanding common factors contributing to sexually motivated offences.

Part II: Summary

Part II focuses on sexual regulation skills and psychosexual education relevant to healthy sexuality and wellbeing. Specifically, this module encourages clients to consider their sexual schemas and how to create healthier sexual thoughts and behaviors. They will learn skills such as CALM and CLASP to regulate and stop deviant sexual fantasies and arousal. Furthermore, clients will learn about the dynamic and acute risk factors associated with reoffending, and will identify their personal risk factors. Finally, clients will gain a deeper understanding of their offense(s) by analyzing their own biological, psychological, and social vulnerabilities that led to the offense(s) through completion of the Offense Staircase.

Part III: Summary

Part III focuses on interpersonal relationships and interpersonal effectiveness skills. Many people who have committed sexually motivated offenses struggle with interpersonal relationships—both sexual and platonic. Part III encourages clients to critically reflect upon their relationships in order to identify, develop, and maintain their support system(s); and consider the issues that led to problematic relationships in their lives. This section addresses important aspects of creating and maintaining healthy relationships with others, including mindful communication, setting and respecting boundaries, identifying barriers to intimate partner relationships, and empathy. In addition, clients will learn the specific interpersonal effectiveness skills DEAR MAN and GIVE FAST, to aid them in creating and maintaining prosocial relationships.

Part IV: Summary

Part IV addresses emotional regulation. Emotional challenges such as dysregulation or overregulation are typically implicated in sexual offending. Emotion regulation and management skills have been shown to decrease sexual, general, and violent reoffending. In this section, clients will acknowledge and identify their feelings; begin to understand how their emotions, and wise and risky thoughts, are intertwined with their behavior; and learn to tolerate long-term pain and vulnerabilities through radical acceptance.

Part V: Summary

Part V focuses on distress tolerance, or learning how to use healthy and effective coping skills in distressing situations. The purpose of learning skills such as STOP, CABB, Wise Mind ACCEPTS, self-soothing, and RAW PAR is to help clients effectively cope with an immediate crisis without increasing suffering. These skills are not for long-term use, because they are only meant to help when we are faced with *immediate* threats. Clients will learn how to differentiate between life-threatening situations and perceived immediate threats, as well as how to use their mindfulness skills to cope in these situations. The module concludes with a detailed (re)lapse prevention plan that clients will complete to continue using their skills to avoid a lapse, and ultimately reoffense.

Weekly Sessions: Outline

- Mindfulness exercise (5–10 minutes).
- Check-in: Review homework and diary cards as a group (approximately 45 minutes). Ask each participant to discuss their assignments. What did they notice as they were completing the assignments? What overlaps stuck out to them? What can they do to navigate their inner and interpersonal challenges when they arise and get to a state of wise mind?

- Five to 10-minute break.
- Introduce weekly topic and skills (50–60 minutes).

Notes

1 See Tomlinson (2018).
2 Haktanır & Callender (2020).
3 Ciesinski, Sorgi-Wilson, Cheung, Chen & McCloskey (2022).
4 Harned et al. (2012).
5 Feigenbaum, Fonagy, Pilling, Jones, Wildgoose, & Bebbington (2012); Shelton, Sampl, Kesten, Zhang, & Trestman (2009).
6 Rosenfeld, Galietta, Foellmi, Coupland, Turner, Stern, Wijetunga, Gerbrandij, & Ivanoff (2019).
7 McCann, Ball, & Ivanoff (2000).
8 Wetterborg, Delhbombom, Långström, Andersson, Fruzzetti, & Enebrink (2020).
9 McCann et al. (2000).
10 Dingfelder (2004).
11 See Sakdalan & Gupta (2014); Shingler (2004); Vess, (2008).
12 See Sakdalan, Shaw, & Collier (2010); Shingler (2004).
13 See Craig, Browne, & Beech (2008); Hanson & Morton-Bourgon (2005).
14 Ward & Stewart (2003); Ward & Gannon (2006).
15 Ward and Gannon (2006) refer to the goals for creating a good life as "primary/secondary goods"; whereas Linehan (1993, 2015) discusses the importance of teaching skillful means and dialectics to create a life worth living.
16 McCann, Ivanoff, Schmidt, & Beach (2007).
17 Tomlinson (2018).
18 Arbanas (2022).
19 Levenson, Willis, & Prescott (2014); Reavis, Looman, Franco, & Rojas (2013).
20 P. 3.
21 Sakdalan and Gupta (2014).
22 Hanson, & Morton-Bourgon (2005); Hanson & Bussière (1998); Hanson & Harris (2000).
23 Bonta & Andrews (2007).
24 According to Proliteracy (2023), "75% of state incarcerated individuals did not complete high school or can be classified as low literate."
25 Linehan (1993).
26 Andrews, Bonta, & Hodge (1990).
27 Smid, Kamphuis, Weaver, & Verbruggen (2015).
28 CSC (2009). For further discussion about treatment dosage for men who have committed sexual offences, see Day, Ross, Casey, Vess, Johns, & Hobbs (2019); and Hanson & Yates (2013).

References

Andrews D. A., Bonta J., & Hoge R. D. (1990). Classification for effective rehabilitation: Rediscovering psychology. *Criminal Justice and Behavior, 17*(1), 19–52. https://doi.org/10.1177/0093854890017001004

Arbanas G. (2022). Personality disorders in sex offenders, compared to offenders of other crimes. *The Journal of Sexual Medicine, 19*(11). https://doi.org/10.1016/j.jsxm.2022.08.022

Bonta J., & Andrews D. A. (2007). *Risk-Need-Responsivity Model for Offender Assessment and Rehabilitation* (No. PS3-1/2007-6) (pp. 1–22). Ottawa, ON: Public Safety Canada.

Ciesinski N. K., Sorgi-Wilson K. M., Cheung J.C., Chen E. Y., McCloskey M. S. (2022). The effect of dialectical behavior therapy on anger and aggressive behavior: A systematic review with meta-analysis. *Behaviour Research and Therapy*, (154), 104122. https://doi.org/10.1016/j.brat.2022.104122

Correctional Service Canada. (2009). *Correctional Program Descriptions*. http://www.csc-scc.gc.ca/text/pa/cop-prog/cp-eval-eng.html

Craig L. A., Browne K. D., & Beech A. R. (2008). Assessing risk in sex offenders: A practitioner's guide. Chichester: John Wiley & Sons Ltd. https://doi.org/10.1002/9780470773208

Day A., Ross S., Casey S., Vess J., Johns D., & Hobbs G. (2019). The intensity and timing of sex offender treatment. *Sexual Abuse, 31*(4), 397–409. https://doi.org/10.1177/1079063217745069

Dingfelder S. F. (2004). Treatment for the 'untreatable'. *Monitor on Psychology, 35*(3), 46. https://www.apa.org/monitor/mar04/treatment.html

Feigenbaum J. D., Fonagy P., Pilling S., Jones A., Wildgoose A., & Bebbington P. E. (2012). A real-world study of the effectiveness of DBT in the UK National Health Service. *The British Journal of Clinical Psychology, 51*(2), 121–141. https://doi.org/10.1111/j.2044-8260.2011.02017

Haktanır A., & Callender K. A. (2020). Meta-analysis of dialectical behavior therapy (DBT) for treating substance use. *Research on Education and Psychology, 4*(Special Issue), 74–87.

Harned M. S., Korslund K. E., Foa E. B., & Linehan M. M. (2012). Treating PTSD in suicidal and self-injuring women with borderline personality disorder: Development and preliminary evaluation of a Dialectical Behavior Therapy Prolonged Exposure Protocol. *Behaviour Research and Therapy, 50*(6), 381–386. https://doi.org/10.1016/j.brat.2012.02.011

Hanson R. K., & Harris A. J. R. (2000). Where should we intervene? Dynamic predictors of sexual assault recidivism. *Criminal Justice and Behavior, 27*(1), 6–35. https://doi.org/10.1177/0093854800027001002

Hanson R. K., & Bussière M. T. (1998). Predicting relapse: A meta-analysis of sexual offender recidivism studies. *Journal of Consulting and Clinical Psychology, 66*(2), 348–362. https://doi.org/10.1037/0022-006X.66.2.348

Levenson, J. S., & Willis, G. M. (2014). Trauma-informed care with sexual offenders. In Carich M. S., & Mussack S. E. *The Safer Society Handbook of Sexual Abuser Assessment and Treatment* (pp 243–269). Brandon, VT: Safer Society Press.

Levins R., & Lewontin R. (1985). *The Dialectical Biologist*. Cambridge, MA: Harvard University Press.

Linehan M. M. (2015). Skills Training Manual (2nd ed.). New York: Guilford Press.

Linehan M. M (1993). *Cognitive-Behavioral Treatment of Borderline Personality Disorder*. New York: Guilford Publications.

Hanson R. K & Yates, P. (2013). Psychological treatment of sex offenders. *Current Psychiatry Reports, (15)*348. https://doi.org/10.1007/s11920-012-0348

Hanson R. K., & Morton-Bourgon K. E. (2005). The characteristics of persistent sexual offenders: A meta-analysis of recidivism studies. *Journal of Consulting and Clinical Psychology, 73*(6), 1154–1163. https://doi.org/10.1037/0022-006X.73.6.1154

McCann R. A., Ball E. M., & Ivanoff A. (2000). DBT with an inpatient forensic population: The CMHIP forensic model. *Cognitive and Behavioral Practice, 7*(4), 447–456. https://doi.org/10.1016/S1077-7229(00)80056-5

McCann R. A., Ivanoff A. Schmidt H., & Beach B. (2007). Implementing dialectical behavior therapy in residential forensic settings with adults and juveniles. In Dimeff L. & Koerner K. (eds.), *Dialectical Behavior Therapy in Clinical Practice: Applications across Disorders and Settings* (pp.112–146). New York: Guilford Press.

Proliteracy (2023). *U.S. Adult Literacy Facts*. https://www.proliteracy.org/Adult-Literacy-Facts

Reavis J. A., Looman J., Franco K. A., & Rojas, B. (2013). Adverse childhood experiences and adult criminality: How long must we live before we possess our own lives? *The Permanente Journal, 17*(2), 44–48. https://doi.org/10.7812/TPP/12-072

Rosenfeld B., Galietta M., Foellmi M., Coupland S., Turner Z., Stern S., Wijetunga C., Gerbrandij J., & Ivanoff A. (2019). Dialectical behavior therapy (DBT) for the treatment of stalking offenders: A randomized controlled study. *Law and Human Behavior, 43*(4), 319–328. https://doi.org/10.1037/lhb0000336

Sakdalan J. A. & Gupta, R. (2014). Wise mind–risky mind: A reconceptualisation of dialectical behaviour therapy concepts and its application to sexual offender treatment. *Journal of Sexual Aggression, 20*(1), 110–120. https://.doi.10.1080/13552600.2012.723357

Sakdalan J. A., Shaw J., & Collier V. (2010). Staying in the here-and-now: A pilot study on the use of dialectical behaviour therapy group skills training for forensic clients with intellectual disability. *Journal of Intellectual Disability Research, 54*(6), 568–572. https://doi.org/10.1111/j.1365-2788.2010.01274.x

Shelton D., Sampl S., Kesten K. L., Zhang W., & Trestman R. L. (2009). Treatment of impulsive aggression in correctional settings. *Behavioral Sciences & the Law, 27*(5), 787–800. https://doi.org/10.1002/bsl.889

Shingler J. (2004). What sex offender treatment can learn from dialectical behavior therapy. *Journal of Offender Rehabilitation, 39*(4), 69–86. http://doi.org/10.1300/J076v39n04_05

Smid W. J., Kamphuis J. H., Wever E. C., & Verbruggen M. C. (2015). Risk levels, treatment duration, and drop out in a clinically composed outpatient sex offender treatment group. *Journal of Interpersonal Violence, 30*(5), 727–743. https://doi.org/10.1177/0886260514536276

Tomlinson M. F. (2018). A theoretical and empirical review of dialectical behavior therapy within forensic psychiatric and correctional settings worldwide. *The International Journal of Forensic Mental Health, 17*(1), 72–95. https://doi.org/10.1080/14999013.2017.1416003

Vess J. (2008). Risk formulation with sex offenders: Integrating functional analysis and actuarial measures. *Journal of Behavior Analysis of Offender and Victim Treatment Prevention, 1*(4), 29-24.

Ward T. (2002). The management of risk and the design of good lives. *Australian Psychologist, 37*, 172–179.

Ward T., & Stewart C.A. (2003). The treatment of sex offenders: Risk management and good lives. *Professional Psychology Research and Practice, 34*(4), 353–360. https://doi.org/10.1037/0735-7028.34.4.353

Ward T., & Gannon T.A. (2006). Rehabilitation, etiology, and self-regulation: The comprehensive good lives model of treatment for sexual offenders. *Aggression and Violent Behavior, 11*(1), 77–94. https://doi.org/10.1016/j.avb.2005.06.001

Wetterborg D., Dehlbom P., Långström N., Andersson G., Fruzzetti A.E., Enebrink P. (2020). Dialectical behavior therapy for men with borderline personality disorder and antisocial behavior: A clinical trial. *Journal of Personality Disorders, 34*(1), 22–39. http://doi.org/10.1521/pedi_2018_32_379

Part I

Introduction to Skills Training and Mindfulness

An Overview of DBT   1

Programming

Dialectical behavior therapy (DBT) encompasses a comprehensive set of goals aimed at empowering clients to improve their lives. First, it helps clients learn new ways of handling their thoughts, emotions, and behaviors by teaching them useful skills to implement in their lives. Second, it helps clients stay motivated and involved in treatment. Third, it ensures that the skills clients learn in therapy are applied to their daily lives and aid clients in making positive changes. Fourth, it reinforces the therapist's motivation to continue to provide treatment, especially for high-risk and high-needs clients. Finally, it aids clients in making changes in their surroundings so they can understand the dialectics, or tension, between wise and risky thoughts, feelings, and behavior; and can use their skills effectively in various situations.

To effectively realize these objectives, DBT employs four key components designed to assist clients in building a wise life: individual therapy, group skills training, telephone consultation, and the therapist consultation group.

Individual Therapy

In DBT, the roles of the individual therapist and the skills trainer are both crucial and complementary. They must work together to provide a comprehensive treatment approach. The individual therapist focuses on the client's specific needs by providing individualized, weekly therapy, addressing complex issues,

DOI: 10.4324/9781003451099-3

and implementing crisis intervention and safety planning. The therapist is responsible for assessing and identifying the client's treatment targets and working with the client to collaboratively develop an individualized treatment plan. Further, by providing a supportive and validating environment, the therapist helps facilitate change by "fold[ing] the skills training into the ongoing psychotherapy" [1] to address cognitive distortions, problem behaviors and emotional dysregulation, reinforcing skills practice, and working on effective coping mechanisms.

Skills Training

While the individual therapist focuses on the client's specific needs and facilitates change through personalized therapy, the skills trainer plays a vital role in teaching and reinforcing skills within the group setting. The skills trainer's role is a fundamental component of treatment that is essential for successful implementation of DBT. The role of the skills trainer includes the following:

- Facilitating weekly DBT skills training group by providing psycho-education, helpful examples, and practical exercises to help clients learn and practice skills effectively.
- Aiding clients in generalizing the skills to their everyday lives by encouraging them to use real-life situations where they can implement their skills. The skills trainer then provides guidance on implementing and/or adapting the skills.
- Using positive reinforcement and motivation to support and maintain client engagement, and commitment to, and practice of skills training.

Telephone Consultation

Telephone coaching or consultation plays an important role in DBT by providing clients with support and guidance outside of therapy through phone calls. There are three key reasons why telephone coaching is an important component of DBT. First, telephone consultations help clients practice effective communication when seeking assistance. Whether the client tends to refrain from asking for help because of fear, guilt, or shame, or is aggressive and demanding when asking for help, phone consultations allow the therapist to work with the client to use effective means of communication to ask for support. Second, providing phone consultations aids in skill application and generalization to clients' daily lives. It not only reinforces the application of skills outside of therapy, but also allows clients to contact their therapists for guidance and practical suggestions when they feel stuck, or when a crisis arises. Lastly, phone consultations help strengthen the therapeutic relationship between client and therapist by fostering accessibility, trust, and a sense of support between therapy sessions, which can promote treatment engagement and motivation.

Telephone consultations are not the appropriate time to conduct therapy, but rather involve coaching clients who are experiencing a crisis situation. In other words, the phone consultation should be used to help a client get through a difficult situation effectively; the situation can then be discussed and analyzed in greater depth during the next individual session. Some of your clients may regularly experience crisis situations; or you may feel your client is "taking advantage" of you. I set boundaries for telephone consultations with clients when they begin treatment. For example, I allow my clients to text me when they have used their skills outside of treatment or have accomplished a major goal. These texts are met with positive reinforcement. They are also allowed to text if something has come up and they are unable to make it to individual or group therapy that week, or if they have a quick question. I encourage clients to call me if:

- They are having thoughts of harming themselves.
- They are having thoughts of harming someone else.
- They are experiencing a real or perceived crisis situation and need skills coaching.

Additionally, I will sometimes initiate phone contact with clients to "check in" if they were struggling with negative emotions during a treatment session, or are experiencing a major life transition.

Telephone coaching poses a challenge if you work in a correctional setting. If this is the case, working with and encouraging correctional officers to coach clients experiencing a crisis is helpful.[2] Of course, not all correctional officers are "on board" with "providing treatment" to offenders due to personal beliefs or a lack of time/resources. It is important to facilitate a respectful and helpful relationship with correctional staff to encourage them to "buy into" the treatment. You may be able to "sell" the treatment by letting them know that you have mutual goals related to prison safety and security, and that treatment is effective in reducing behavioral disruptions, which leads to decreased strain on correctional staff.[3] Additionally, you may opt to employ DEAR MAN with staff to reinforce a plan that will be mutually beneficial (see Chapter 10 for an explanation of DEAR MAN skills).

Case Consultation for Therapists

Working with individuals who have committed sexual offenses is stressful and can be frustrating. Some treatment providers internalize their frustration as fear or shock, which has the tendency to surface as iatrogenic behaviors during treatment or toward the client, such as "victim blaming."[4] As clinicians, we have an ethical obligation to appropriately address maladaptive emotions or behaviors that may arise during treatment. As such, case consultation meetings for therapists are a crucial component of working with sex offenders.[5] The consultation group serves as both support and supervision for the clinician in order to ensure they effectively implement the principles and strategies of DBT, remain engaged in treatment, and effectively address therapy-interfering behaviors that may arise during treatment. Key components of the therapist consultation group include enhancing the clinician's ability to provide effective DBT, and skills development through case consultation.

Therapist Characteristics

DBT addresses the importance of therapist characteristics and skills by outlining syntheses of dialectical opposites. These characteristics allow the therapist to create a safe and supportive therapeutic environment while responding to the client's needs with empathy and understanding. It is crucial that DBT therapists learn to balance these characteristics to provide effective, compassionate, trauma-informed care to their clients.[6] In addition, therapists may engage in therapy-interfering behaviors that reduce the efficacy of treatment and may even cause the client distress if there is an imbalance between the way each dialectical dimension is addressed. The purpose of DBT consultation groups is, in part, to help the clinician identify and address their own therapy-interfering behaviors.

The first dimension, "acceptance vs. change," means that the therapist must be able to both accept the client's current reality (i.e., "radical acceptance") *and* encourage change. In DBT, clients work toward accepting their thoughts and emotions as they are in the moment, while simultaneously working to change the patterns or behaviors that result from negative thoughts or emotional dysregulation. This requires the therapist to teach the client new behavioral skills to help them live a more effective life while remaining empathic to their current experience. Imbalance in this domain refers to a therapist's tendency to rely too heavily on either accepting the client as they are or pushing too hard for change. Too much focus on acceptance can prevent a client from making necessary changes in their lives, whereas too much focus on change can create client resistance.

The second dimension is that of "unwavering centeredness vs. compassionate flexibility." This refers to the therapist's ability to maintain a non-judgmental, non-reactive stance in the face of a client's intense emotional outburst(s) and problematic or therapy-interfering behaviors, while being responsive to the client's needs—all without compromising structure or consistency in the therapeutic process. A balance of these characteristics helps the therapist build a positive therapeutic alliance without colluding with the client. An imbalance, however, can lead a client to resist a therapist whom they consider to be too rigid, or can destabilize the structure of treatment and reduce expectations of client accountability.

The third dimension involves creating a synthesis between the dimensions of being "nurturing vs. benevolently demanding." On one hand, the therapist must be able to create a safe and supportive environment for the client to explore his emotions and experiences. Nurturing helps clients feel validated, understood, and respected. On the other hand, an effective therapist is one who creates structure and accountability in order to help clients make changes to effectively live a life of meaning. Balancing these characteristics is a crucial component in building and maintaining a positive rapport with your client while pushing them to use skillful means to build a wise life. Again, an imbalance in this dimension can lead to a reduction in client accountability, or place undue pressure on the client to change, thus fostering a sense of inadequacy or stasis.

In addition to the importance of therapist characteristics, it is crucial for the therapist to be mindful and establish clear agreements to which they will adhere. These agreements include making "every reasonable effort" to assist the client during the course of treatment, as recommended by Linehan; addressing common misconceptions about therapy and the role of the therapist with the client before treatment begins; adhering to ethical behavior and treatment guidelines set by law and their licensing board; establishing guidelines for "personal contact" in terms of how often or when a client can reach out to the therapist; respecting the client's humanity and rights throughout the treatment process; and maintaining confidentiality.

Therapy-Interfering Behaviors

In DBT, there are several client-initiated, therapy-interfering behaviors that can hinder the client's progress and undermine the effectiveness of therapy.

Thus, it is important to identify and address the following types of therapy-interfering behaviors in order to create a more productive and effective therapeutic environment:[7]

- **Nonattentive behaviors** are behaviors indicating a lack of attention or engagement in the treatment process. These can include not participating in group, or appearing uninterested in treatment (e.g., yawning loudly, rolling eyes). These behaviors interfere with therapy because they prevent clients from fully engaging in therapy.
- **Noncollaborative behaviors** are behaviors indicating a client's unwillingness to achieve therapeutic goals. These might include arguing with the therapist, lying, not talking, resisting suggestions or feedback, monopolizing the conversation, or coming in late for treatment each week.
- **Noncompliant behaviors** refer to a client's unwillingness to follow through with treatment and/or supervision expectations. Examples may include not attending treatment, creating a hostile treatment environment, not completing homework or diary cards, or violating conditions of probation or parole.

Therapy-interfering behaviors can be frustrating for the therapist and other group members. During one of the initial individual sessions, it is helpful for the therapist to acknowledge that while they have an obligation to provide the client with the skills, resources, and support necessary to build a wise life, the client *also* has an obligation to the therapist and the group to appropriately engage in treatment and actively use their skills and resources. As a therapist, you have an obligation to use every reasonable effort to provide treatment to your client; however, you do not have an unconditional obligation to continue working with clients who repeatedly violate rules or expectations. Termination of treatment should be used only as a last resort, but clients need to understand from the beginning that this is a possibility.

If a client is engaging in therapy-interfering behaviors, the individual therapist should address this in therapy. A functional analysis of the behavior—such as behavior chain analysis or missing link analysis (see Chapter 2)—is a useful place to start to encourage the client to take a critical look at his behavior and identify and implement skills to work toward living a more effective life.

Therapists are also encouraged to use contingency management based on the principles of operant conditioning. These techniques have been shown to be effective in shaping offender behavior, especially when positive reinforcement such as token economy is used instead of punishment. When implemented swiftly and consistently, positive reinforcement demonstrates encouraging results in shaping desired behaviors, especially among incarcerated populations.[8] However, working in an institutional setting comes with its own unique challenges, and treatment providers' options are limited to following institutional policies and procedures.[9]

Quality-of-Life-Interfering Behaviors

The quality-of-life-interfering behaviors within the context of sexual offending include dynamic acute risk-related areas that should regularly be assessed by treatment providers and community supervision officers. These seven areas have been identified by Fernandez et al. (2015) in the *ACUTE-2007 Coding Manual—Revised*:[10]

- Victim access: The client has increased opportunities to have contact with potential victims.
- Hostility (general): An increase in aggressive behaviors; increased anger toward others, primarily women or authority figures.
- Sexual preoccupation: Increased changes in deviant or non-deviant sexual behavior, thoughts, or fantasies.
- Rejection of supervision: Non-compliance with conditions of supervision.
- Emotional collapse: Recent changes in the offender's emotional state; failure to use prosocial coping skills; increased depression or anxiety; feeling overwhelmed.
- Change in social supports: Loss or perceived loss of prosocial friends or family in the offender's social network; increased contact with antisocial peers or family members; social withdrawal.
- Substance abuse: Likelihood of drug or alcohol abuse since last contact with clinician or community supervision officer

Helping clients create a structured lifestyle can be useful, especially if the client has limited social interactions or a tendency to withdraw.[11] Lack of engagement or decreased engagement with prosocial family, peers, or activities typically leads to changes in an individual's emotional state and thus their use of helpful coping skills. I currently work in an outpatient clinic with individuals who have numerous restrictions placed upon them, such as no Internet access; ankle monitoring devices; housing restrictions, including public and private spaces they must avoid; and people with whom they are not allowed to maintain contact. Many outpatient clients feel a sense of hopelessness because they "can't do anything" while on probation or parole.

As such, I have created and regularly update a board in the group room containing low or no-cost, adult-only, alcohol-free events in the community. I encourage clients to consider attending an event or events and interacting with others. If you are working with institutionalized patients or offenders, this strategy is not possible, of course. In that case, I have encouraged patients and inmates to take advantage of activities to which they do have access, such as walking and other exercise, playing cards or games with others, setting up an art / writing group, or attending religious or spiritual groups.

In addition to addressing quality-of-life-interfering behaviors, it is important also to identify clients' protective factors. Over the last two decades, criminological research has addressed the importance of identifying offenders' protective factors, or factors that mitigate and promote desistance in offending.[12] More recently, scholars and clinicians in the field of sex offender treatment have begun to focus on protective factors in addition to risk factors, to provide a stronger emphasis on strengths-based treatment rather than using the traditional deficits-based model.

In 2007, de Vogel and colleagues developed the Structured Assessment of PROtective Factors (SAPROF) to assess factors supporting desistance from violent offending. Since then, Willis and colleagues have modified the SAPROF to assess protective factors for sexual offenders (2020; SAPROF-SO). "Concerning practice implications, the SAPROF-SO provides a useful clinical and risk management tool that aligns with strength-based approaches to rehabilitation including the Good Lives Model."[13] Specifically, the SAPROF-SO was designed to theoretically align with the assumptions of the Good Lives Model, while also focusing on the desistance and sexual offending research.[14]

Hierarchy of Treatment Targets

Each stage of DBT is part of a larger, structured hierarchy of treatment targets. Treatment targets for therapists working with sex offenders should address dynamic, stable, and acute risk factors for sexual offending.[15] Sakdalan and Gupta (2014) reconceptualized the hierarchy of treatment targets to address the treatment needs of sexual offenders.[16]

Addressing Treatment Target Areas

- **Sexual dysregulation:** Implement skills[17] to address the dangers of sexual preoccupation, using sex for coping, sexual preferences, and access to victims.

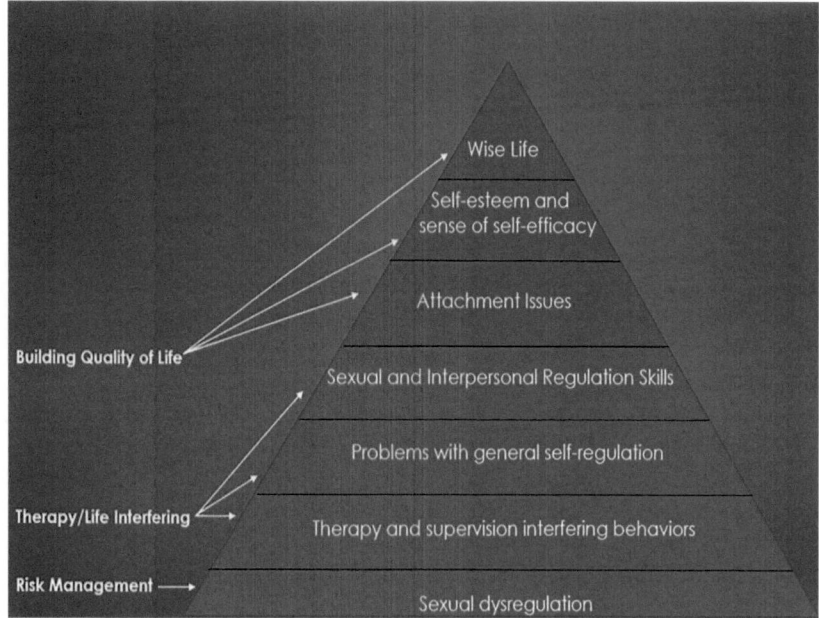

Image 1.1 Sakdalan & Gupta's (2014) reconceptualization of treatment target and needs

- **Therapy and supervision-interfering behaviors:** Address hostility and rejection of supervision.
- **Problems with general self-regulation:** Address problems with affect and emotional regulation such as negative emotionality, substance use, impulsivity, and poor problem-solving skills.
- **Sexual and interpersonal regulation skills:** Address capacity for relationship stability, hostility toward women, emotional identification with children, and general social rejection and/or loneliness.
- **Attachment issues:** Address historical trauma and attachment issues.
- **Problems with general self-esteem and self-efficacy:** Assist the client by setting longer-term goals.
- **Wise life:** Address any other treatment goals or needs necessary to live effectively and maintain a life worth living.

Overall, the purpose of creating and implementing a structured hierarchy is twofold. First, it ensures that the client and clinician are clear and united about specific treatment targets, and can thus work toward goals. Second, it assists clinicians in ensuring consistency throughout treatment.

Notes

1 Linehan (1993; p. 103).
2 See Sampl, Wakai, & Trestman (2010; p. 116) for a discussion about recommendations to increase correctional staff receptivity to treatment.
3 Applebaum, Hickey, & Packer (2001).
4 Linehan (1993; 2015).
5 Levenson & Willis (2014).
6 Levenson, Willis, & Prescott (2017); Levenson, Willis, & Prescott (2016); Levenson & Willis (2014).
7 Linehan (1993; pp. 132–134).
8 See Gendreau, Listwan, & Kuhns (2011).
9 Sampl, Wakai, & Trestman (2010) address potential issues that can arise when working within institutional settings, such as enhancing correctional support of, or "buy-in" to, programming; restrictions on material allowed to enter the facility; treatment tools that may not be provided within the setting; and working around potential inmate movement restrictions.
10 For a more detailed description and scoring of acute risk factors, see Fernandez, Gotch, Hanson, and A. J. R. Harris (2015).
11 Please see Handout 18.1: My Relapse Prevention Plan.
12 For example, see Herrenkohl et al. (2003), and de Vogel, de Ruiter, Bouman, & de Vries Robbé (2009, 2012).
13 P. 1463. For further discussion of SAPROF-SO, items, domains, and theoretical alignment see Willis, Kelley, & Thornton (2020)
14 Ward & Gannon (2006).
15 See Brankley, Helmus, & Hanson (2017); Fernandez, A. J. R. Harris, Hanson, & Sparks (2014).
16 Pp. 112–113.
17 Ward & Stewart; (2003); Ward & Gannon (2006)

References

Appelbaum K. L., Hickey J. M., & Packer I. (2001). The role of correctional officers in multidisciplinary mental health care in prisons. *Psychiatric Services (Washington, D.C.)*, *52*(10), 1343–1347. https://doi.org/10.1176/appi.ps.52.10.1343

Brankley A. E., Helmus L. M., & Hanson R. K. (2017). *STABLE-2007 Evaluator Workbook:* Updated recidivism rates (includes combinations with Static-99R, Static-2002R, and Risk Matrix 2000). Unpublished report, Public Safety Canada, Ottawa, Ontario.

de Vogel V., de Ruiter C., Bouman Y., & de Vries Robbé M. (2009). *SAPROF: Guidelines for the Assessment of Protective Factors for Violence Risk* (English version). Utrecht, Netherlands: Forum Educatief.

de Vogel V., de Ruiter C., Bouman Y., & de Vries Robbé M. (2012). *SAPROF: Guidelines for the Assessment of Protective Factors for Violence Risk* (2nd ed.). Utrecht, Netherlands: De Forensische Zorgspecialisten.

de Vries Robbe M., Mann R. E., Maruna S. & Thornton D. (2015). An exploration of protective factors supporting desistance from sexual offending. *Sexual Abuse*, 27(1), 16–33. https://doi:10.1177/1079063214547582

Fernandez Y., Gotch K. R., Hanson R.K., & Harris A. J. R. (2015). *ACUTE-2007 Coding Manual—Revised*. Unpublished report. Ottawa, ON: Public Safety Canada.

Fernandez Y., Harris A. J. R., Hanson R. K., Sparks J. (2014). *STABLE-2007 Coding Manual—Revised 2014*. Unpublished report. Ottawa, ON: Public Safety Canada.

Gendreau P., Listwan S. J., & Kuhns J. B. (2011). *Managing Prisons Effectively: The Potential of Contingency Management Programs*. https://www.publicsafety.gc.ca/cnt/rsrcs/pblctns/2011-04-mp/2011-04-mp-eng.pdf

Herrenkohl T. I., Hill K. G., Chung I. J., Guo J., Abbott R. D., & Hawkins J. D. (2003). Protective factors against serious violent behavior in adolescence: A prospective study of aggressive children. *Social Work Research*, 27, 179–191. doi:10.1093/swr/27.3.179

Levenson J. S., Willis G. M., & Prescott D. S. (2016). Adverse childhood experiences in the lives of male sex offenders: Implications for trauma-informed care. *Sexual Abuse* 28(4), 340–359. https://doi.org/10.1177/1079063214535819

Levenson J. S., Willis G. M., & Prescott D. S. (2017). *Trauma-Informed Care: Transforming Treatment for People who Sexually Abuse*. Safer Society Press.

Levenson J. S., & Willis G. M. (2014). Trauma-informed care with sexual offenders. In Carich M. S., & Mussack S. E. (eds.) *The Safer Society Handbook of Sexual Abuser Assessment and Treatment* (pp. 243–269). Brandon, VT: Safer Society Press.

Linehan M. M (1993). *Cognitive-Behavioral Treatment of Borderline Personality Disorder*. New York: Guilford Publications.

Sakdalan J. A., & Gupta, R. (2014). Wise mind—risky mind: A reconceptualisation of dialectical behaviour therapy concepts and its application to sexual offender treatment. *Journal of Sexual Aggression*, 20(1), 110–120. https://doi.org/10.1080/13552600.2012.724457

Sampl S., Wakai S., & Trestman R. L. (2010). Translating evidence-based practices from community to corrections: An example of implementing DBT-CM. *The Journal of Behavior Analysis of Offender and Victim Treatment and Prevention*, 2(2), 114–123. https://doi.org/10.1037/h0100463

Ward T., & Keenan T. (1999). Child molesters' implicit theories. *Journal of Interpersonal Violence*, 14(8), 821–838. https://doi.org/10.1177/088626099014008003

Ward T., & Gannon T. A. (2006). Rehabilitation, etiology, and self-regulation: The comprehensive Good Lives Model of treatment for sexual offenders. *Aggression and Violent Behavior*, 11(1), 77–94. https://doi.org/10.1016/j.avb.2005.06.001

Willis G. M., Kelley S. M., & Thornton, D. (2020). Are protective factors valid constructs? Interrater reliability and construct validity of proposed protective factors against sexual reoffending. *Criminal Justice and Behavior*, 47(11), 1448–1467. https://doi.org/10.1177/0093854820941039

Preparing Your Client for DBT Skills Training

2

Most or all our clients are in treatment because it has been mandated by the court. Many clients do not want to be in treatment, or do not believe they need it. As clinicians, it is important to acknowledge that few people, in any setting, are immediately driven to participate in an activity, event, or treatment that is forced upon them. How can we realistically expect initial "treatment compliance" and a positive attitude toward treatment when the motivation to complete programming is initially extrinsic? The answer is: we cannot. While research has shown that extrinsic motivation can create a foundation for future change, self-determination theory posits that people are inherently driven to achieve growth. Intrinsic motivation is thus more effective for engaging in and maintaining change over time. [1] In other words, our goal as clinicians is to work with our clients to help facilitate intrinsic motivation. Of course, this is easier said than done.

The Good Lives Model is premised on this idea that an individual's goals in life are driven by the desire to achieve universal *primary human goods* (PHGs), which necessarily have intrinsic value.[2] Research about sexually motivated offenders and motivation to change has demonstrated that clients are more likely to gain intrinsic motivation when the clinician works *with* them in setting goals to meet their PHGs in a prosocial manner, rather than setting goals *for* them.[3] To this end, it is the clinician's role to assist the client in developing treatment goals that align with the individual's PHGs, and their conceptualization of living a wise life—something that should occur first in the client's individual sessions and guide clients throughout the course of treatment.

DOI: 10.4324/9781003451099-4

The therapeutic relationship between therapist and client is critical in terms of achieving treatment adherence and positive outcomes in therapy, as demonstrated by research on the therapeutic alliance in sex offender treatment[4] and dialectical behavior therapy (DBT) for borderline personality disorder.[5] The therapeutic relationship is particularly important in DBT because the treatment involves challenging and intensive interventions. In line with best practice guidelines in treatment, therapists who can build a positive therapeutic alliance with their client are more likely to see more favorable outcomes from treatment. Clinicians will be hard pressed to build a relationship with their clients if they tend to use a confrontational, or adversarial approach.[6] Picture someone dictating what you "need" to focus on in your life, "should" address, or "must stop" doing. This style of communication hinders the development of a supportive and trusting relationship between the client and clinician. Moreover, it is important to empathize with and validate the emotional impact on your clients, who know that they are not permitted to participate in sexual activities that arouse them, or engage in sexual activity with individuals to whom they are attracted. Try to put yourself in their shoes, confronted with the reality of being told that your desires and inclinations are not only unacceptable, but illegal.

Linehan recommends that the foundation of DBT treatment be built on an agreement that suicide is not an acceptable option when striving to build an offense-free life. In the case of sex offender treatment, the therapist and client enter into an agreement that engaging in non-consensual sexual behavior is unacceptable and will not be tolerated within the treatment program. This agreement does not require offenders who deny their offense to have complete insight into their actions, as many offenders initially lack this awareness. Instead, it simply acknowledges that such behavior is incompatible with the pursuit of living a wise life.

Furthermore, creating a strong therapeutic alliance with the client helps practitioners assess and work with the client toward treatment readiness. Although there is a lack of consensus regarding the construct of "treatment readiness" within the academic and therapeutic communities, [7] assisting a client with treatment readiness when they lack motivation for change can be challenging. During the introductory individual sessions, it is crucial that the clinician immediately begin working on the therapeutic alliance by engaging the client through motivational interviewing in order to increase their intrinsic motivation to actively engage in treatment. Consider the following motivational interviewing technique using DBT wording:

CLIENT: I don't even know why I'm here. I'm not a sex offender and I didn't do what they are saying I did.

CLINICIAN: And what do they say you did?

CLIENT: Molesting my 10-year-old niece and one of her friends. The friend's mom called the cops on me. I was babysitting and the girls asked me to play "house" with them. That's all I did!

CLINICIAN: You were just playing house with the girls because they asked you to join in; so why do you think the mother called the cops and reported that you had molested them?

CLIENT: I have no idea. She must hate men and convinced her daughter that I was some kind of predator. Then she had her daughter convince my niece! Now I can't even spend time with my family if girls under the age of 18 are present.

CLINICIAN: I understand that you do not think you need treatment because you did not commit the offense you were charged with. So, moving forward, let's address issues that might lead someone to accuse you of touching minors in a sexual way to make sure something like this never happens to you again.

CLIENT: It won't! I will never go near a kid again. Hell, I just won't leave my house or talk to anyone.

CLINICIAN: I'm not so sure that that is the most effective method for reaching your goals. Maybe we can come up with some other options that will allow you to live a wise life and avoid the possibility of future accusations.

CLIENT: Whatever.

CLINICIAN: Before we do that, however, I would like to begin our work together by making an agreement that touching minors in a sexual way [for other types of offenses you can use the following: "touching someone in a sexual way without their consent"; "viewing images of naked children online"; "talking to minors online"; "exposing genitals in public," etc.] is unacceptable.

CLIENT: Of course it's wrong. Those people are sickos; but I'm not one of them. I would never hurt a child.

CLINICIAN: That's good to hear! You're in a challenging legal situation right now and things must feel pretty daunting. What would a wise life look like to you?

This agreement serves as the basis for the treatment contract and the development of goals to build a life worth living.

Prior to placement in a skills group, DBT requires that clinicians meet individually with prospective clients for four or five sessions to begin to create a therapeutic alliance, orient the client to treatment expectations, obtain informed consent, make an agreement with the client that engaging in illegal sexual behavior is unacceptable, sign a contract for treatment, and help the client identify areas in their lives that have precluded them from living a life worth living, regardless of whether the client is willing to admit their offense.[8] By ensuring treatment readiness in this way, therapists can help set up their clients for success and increase the likelihood of treatment engagement and thus positive treatment outcomes.

Living a "Wise Life"

The central goal of treatment in DBT is to help clients build a life (more) worth living (see Handout 2.1), or a "wise life."[9] Living a wise life involves developing and maintaining a fulfilling and meaningful existence, leading to a reduction in overall suffering. In DBT, it is important to empower your clients by recognizing that they possess the knowledge of what a meaningful life looks like to them. Thus, be sure to explain to your clients that they are responsible for envisioning what this looks like to them, and for establishing goals that are personally meaningful for their wellbeing.

Ask your client to complete Handout 2.1: Living a Wise Life. Encourage clients to be as detailed as possible, and to describe what a better life—or a life worth living—would look like. I have found that clients tend to be vague. For example, they often say, "To be happy," or "To have a job I like." Once they have completed the activity, the client will read his list to the individual therapist. This is important in order to get to know the client better and, most importantly, to tailor treatment to each person using a strengths-based approach.[10]

Why "Skills Training?"

Skills Trainer: Explain that clients will also complete a homework assignment regarding the pros and cons of practicing their skills outside of the group. Then, ask them to weigh the pros and cons of a skills training group. Tell them to write down a description of three to five problem behaviors or situations that they want to change. Next, they should describe their goals to address the behaviors or situations. Finally, they should list the advantages and disadvantages of practicing their skills daily. You will review this assignment next week via group discussion.

Emotions

One crucial component of DBT is the therapist's use of validation. Validation should not be confused with collusion, as it requires the therapist to acknowledge the client's feelings within the context of a given situation. This is done in three ways. First, the therapist actively observes and acknowledges the client's experiences, and how those experiences have influenced current thoughts, feelings, and behaviors. Second, the therapist engages in reflection by empathically mirroring the client's feelings, thoughts, behaviors, and assumptions back to them. A fundamental assumption in DBT is that the client is doing their best to navigate the present moment; though it does not imply that their cognitive, emotional, or behavioral response is helpful or effective. Instead, it signifies that their response is understandable given the context of their experiences. Lastly, the therapist employs direct validation, whereby the client is rewarded or praised for making improvements in their cognitive schema, and for adopting skillful and effective behavior in a challenging situation.

Skills Trainer:

Identifying our feelings is an important component of treatment. Being able to recognize and express our feelings not only makes us more aware of our experiences, but also helps us develop strategies to address intense emotions, reduce acting on these emotions impulsively, and better communicate with others. We experience two types of emotions: primary and secondary.

Primary emotions are universal, and are our most basic emotions. We experience these emotions automatically in response to something we perceive as positive or negative. However, these feelings range in intensity and are often fleeting. Primary emotions include happiness, sadness, fear, anger, disgust, and surprise.

Secondary emotions, on the other hand, are a response to your primary emotion. You can think about primary and secondary emotions as a dandelion with the white fuzzy sphere on top. Once the wind blows, the fuzz flies off the flower stem in different directions. In this analogy, the fuzz on top of the dandelion represents the primary emotion; but as soon as the wind blows, the fuzz—your secondary emotions—unscramble. In other words, your primary emotion is broken up into many other emotions that are easier to address in the moment.

For example, Andrew's partner yells at him for not cleaning the house on Saturday. In addition to cleaning the house, Andrew was supposed to buy groceries, buy a new pair of pants, and go to a job interview. Andrew forgot to clean the house because he was busy doing other tasks. Therefore, he gets angry at his partner because they obviously do not understand how much he had to do that day. He acknowledges the initial feeling of anger but struggles to identify other feelings associated with anger, such as frustration, hurt, and rejection. Andrew—like most people—has trouble teasing apart and identifying his secondary emotions, and is adamant that he is angry. It is important for Andrew to be able to identify the emotions that are secondary to his anger so that he can effectively communicate how he is feeling to his partner.

The following are a few questions that you can ask yourself to identify whether you are experiencing a primary or secondary emotion:

- *Primary:*
  - *"Am I experiencing an emotion directly related to a situation or event?"*
  - *"Once the event ended, did the emotion go away?"*
- *Secondary:*
  - *"Is this emotion becoming more intense?"*
  - *"Am I experiencing this emotion beyond the point when the situation/ event has ended?"*
  - *"Is the emotion difficult to understand?"*

Ask your clients to take out Handout 2.2: The Feeling Wheel, and review it with them.

Furthermore, inform your clients that each week, they will discuss the top portion of the card with their individual therapist, while both individual and group therapy will cover the bottom section. Be sure to provide clients with a new diary card every week to support consistent tracking and progress.

Daily diary cards are a central tool used in DBT to help individuals track their progress. During your introductory sessions with your clients, explain the purpose of filling out daily diary cards (Handout 2.3). Explain to your clients that the most effective way to track their thoughts, behaviors, and emotions is by writing them down, ensuring that their achievements and challenges during the week are tracked. It is important that clients fill in the diary card each day, so encourage them to keep it in a location where they will not forget about it. Consider suggesting a few suitable places, such as:

- On their nightstand.
- Taped to their bathroom mirror.
- In their wallet.
- Next to their front door.

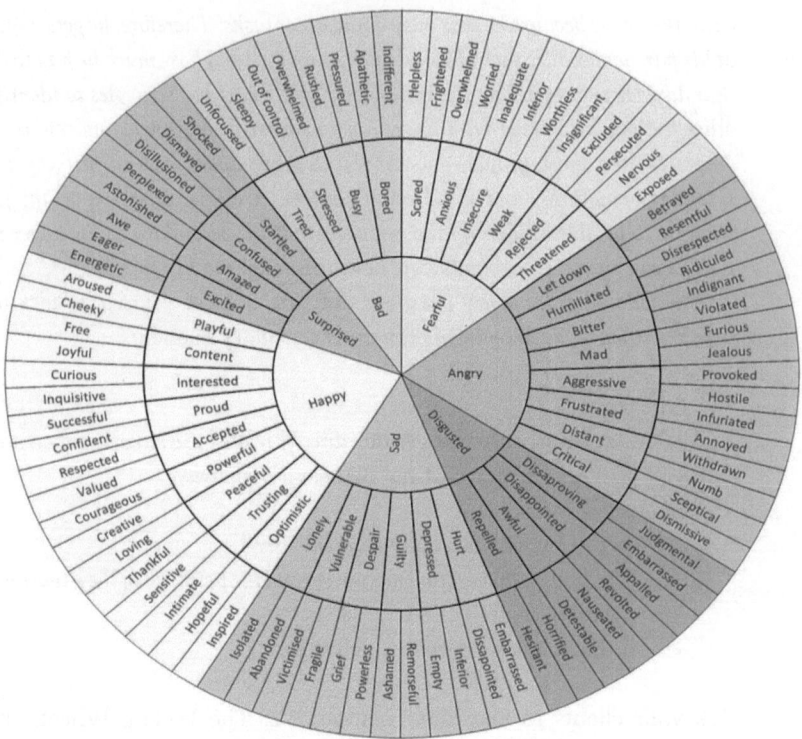

Image 2.1 Feeling Wheel

While this section provides an overview of emotions, a more comprehensive discussion can be found in Part 4 of this book, "Emotion Regulation Skills." The individual therapist may want to initially work with their client on this prior to beginning the group sessions.

Behavior Chain Analysis

Skills Trainer: Ask your client to refer to Handout 2.4: Behavior Chain Analysis and explain the step-by-step process of completing the BCA. Convey the following:

I recognize that it can be challenging to understand why we behave in a certain way, especially when it is unhelpful or illegal. It is often also hard to figure out what factors contributed to the behavior. It is common for individuals to respond with, "I don't know" when asked about the motivations behind their behavior. The purpose of the BCA is to guide you in analyzing the thoughts, behaviors, and emotions that led to your **problem behavior.** *It enables you to understand your vulnerabilities leading up to the problem behavior and the consequences of the behavior, and to practice effective problem solving. Essentially, the BCA assists you in dissecting all the factors that have played a role in your problem behavior(s).*

In the initial sessions, you will ask clients time to complete a BCA about a problem behavior other than their offense (e.g., overeating, substance misuse, yelling, masturbating to fantasies of illegal behavior). This aims to familiarize themselves with the BCA and practice using it before moving forward and analyzing their offense(s). Provide clients with feedback and questions that they may not have considered as they completed their BCA. You might also want to use the BCA with your clients to analyze wise behaviors in order to help them maintain a wise mind, and to reinforce and generalize their skills.

Later in treatment, you will ask your client to complete a BCA about their offense or offenses. If they deny their offense, you can work with them to address a problematic behavior that placed them in the risky situation that ultimately led to their arrest and/or incarceration. You will continue to use the BCA throughout treatment as a tool to help your client address any ineffective or unskillful behavior. This could include lashing out at someone, lying, or allowing themselves to orgasm to a fantasy about an illegal situation, among other things.

Skills Trainer: Ask your client to look at Handout 2.4: Behavior Chain Analysis. Throughout the course of treatment, you will continue to use the BCA to help provide a comprehensive review of all problematic behaviors that arise. This will ensure that clients consistently reflect on and gain insights into their past actions, to foster a deeper understanding of their behavioral patterns and identify progress along the way.

- **Describe the problem behavior:** Explain to your client that they should begin the BCA by describing, in detail, the problem behavior. They should carefully explain what they did, thought, or felt, and rate the severity of the behavior, thought, or feeling on a scale of 1–10 (with 10 being most extreme).
- Examples might include missing treatment; losing their temper with someone (this could include becoming overly angry and ruminating about the situation, or lashing out verbally/physically

at someone); isolating; misusing drugs or alcohol; fantasizing about illegal behavior; or masturbating to fantasies of illegal behavior.

- If the problem behavior is something that they did not do, encourage them to ask themselves whether they:
  - Forgot about it?
  - Stopped thinking about it, and intentionally "forgot" about it?
  - Procrastinated, and never followed through?
  - Refused to do it? If so, how come?
  - Thought about doing it, but decided they would rather not? If so, how come?
- **Describe the prompting event:** The client should be specific about the exact event or situation that led to the problematic thought, feeling, or behavior. In other words, what was happening directly *before* the behavior?
- **Describe the specific vulnerability factors:** What factors led them to be vulnerable to the problem behavior immediately before they did it? Examples might include:
  - A stressful event.
  - An argument with a loved one, or co-worker.
  - Intrusive thoughts.
  - Being isolated from others.
- **Describe the chain of events (links) in detail:** This differs from the prompting event because it includes the thoughts, emotions, and behaviors that occurred as a result of the event. Be sure to have the client explain this in detail and include:
  - Their actions leading up to the problem behavior.
  - Their thoughts about the prompting event. What did they tell themselves?
  - Their feelings about the prompting event.
  - The physical sensations in their body.
  - How "a" led to "b," led to "c," led to "d" (a→b→c→d). Once they have identified the links, suggest they look at them and consider if there are more links—perhaps smaller links—they might not have considered. These should all be included.
- Example: Your client Jordan feels lonely (vulnerability factor) and wants to have a connection with someone. He then thinks, "I feel uncomfortable talking to women" (prompting event). Jordan's fear (of rejection/of having to feel uncomfortable doing what it would take to initiate a connection with a woman) and loneliness lead him to:
  - Think about making physical contact with a woman.

- o   Leave his home.
- o   Walk to the bus station.
- o   Get on the bus.
- o   Rub up against a stranger in order to become aroused.
- These are all examples of the chain of events, or links, between Jordan's prompting event and problem behavior. You can use this example as an opportunity to validate your client's challenges and encouraging them to practice their skills to work on their challenges.
- Describe the consequences of the behavior:
  - o   What was happening while they engaged in the behavior?
  - o   What happened immediately after the behavior?
  - o   What happened later that day or week?
  - o   What were their thoughts about the behavior?
  - o   What were their feelings after engaging in the behavior?
  - o   How did others respond to their behavior?
  - o   What impact did the behavior have on them, others, or their environment?
- **Describe where skillful behavior could have been used at each point in the BCA**: Where could your client have used skillful behavior at each point?
- Example: Jordan's vulnerability is loneliness. Skills he could have used include practicing mindfulness, calling friends or family, or going for a walk. The prompting event is his thought about being uncomfortable (fearful) talking to women. Skills he could have used include calling friends or family, going to a cafe and finding someone to talk to, or searching for a community group where likeminded people participate in specific activities. The links in the chain might include:
  - o   *Thinking about making physical contact with a woman.*
  - o   *Feeling excited about making physical contact with a woman.*
- Skillful behaviors he could use instead include snapping a rubber band on his wrist, smelling ammonia salts, or taking a cold shower.
  - o   *Leaving his home.*
- Skillful behaviors he could use instead include practicing mindfulness, watching television, or calling a family member or friend.
  - o   *Walking to the bus station.*
- Skillful behaviors he could use instead include using STOP skills (see Chapter 16) or problem-solving skills.
  - o   *Getting on the bus.*

- Skillful behaviors he could use instead include using Opposite Action (see Chapter 15).
- **Describe a prevention strategy to reduce vulnerability to engaging in the problem behavior in the future:** Here, it might be helpful for the client to look at their strengths assignment and determine which of their strengths they could use to prevent this situation from happening again. They should explain *how* they will use these strengths in a similar situation.
- **Describe how to repair the consequences of the problem behavior:** The client should answer the following questions:
  - Whom or what did they harm? (Explain how their behavior led to harm.)
  - What is the harm they caused?
  - What actions are needed in order to repair that harm? (Explain how their actions could repair the harm. This does not necessarily mean that someone will forgive them for their actions, but rather that they have openly acknowledged what they have done and are making an effort to correct the behavior.)

Example of a BCA

Gio was 12 months sober, but decided to go to the bar on a Friday evening with a few friends, including Marissa. He was having problems in his marriage and found comfort in his perception that Marissa was flirting with him. This example provides concrete examples of thinking errors and risk factors that led to Gio's initial offense, his relapse from sobriety, and the creation of more interpersonal problems for himself. It is important to understand and intervene during a behavioral lapse in order to avoid a sexual relapse.

- **Behavior:** "I started drinking again and was flirting too much with my friend, Marissa."
- **Vulnerabilities:**
  - "My wife stopped having sex with me and I felt like I deserved a drink or two" (challenges with interpersonal relationships; feelings of loneliness; feelings of rejection; entitlement).
  - "I don't like talking about my emotions, and my wife and I never talk about our relationship" (challenges with interpersonal relationships).
  - "I was horny" (challenges with sexual regulation).

- Prompting event:
  - ○ "I was out at the bar with my friends and drank about six beers that night, but it's not like I was really drunk or anything" (substance use).
  - ○ "This woman was flirting with me" (assumption).
- Links:
  - ○ "I was happy because it was the end of the week and I was out with my friends."
  - ○ "I was upset because my wife stopped having sex with me, which made me feel unappreciated" (interpersonal problems; feelings of rejection).
  - ○ "Marissa has sex with lots of men, so it was obvious that she wanted to sleep with me" (assumption; rose-colored lenses).
- Outcomes of the behavior:
  - ○ "I began masturbating to fantasies of Marissa."
  - ○ "I continued to go out with my friend group and get drunk every weekend to loosen up so I could flirt with Marissa."
  - ○ "I was upset with myself because I was sober for one year before I decided to drink again."
  - ○ "I made Marissa feel uncomfortable."
  - ○ "My friends told me I was acting like a jackass."
  - ○ "My relationship with my wife got worse."
- Skills he could have used during the chain to stop the behavior:
  - ○ Go home after closing time.
  - ○ Not drinking in the first place.
  - ○ Not flirting with other women.

Missing Links Analysis[11]

Skills Trainer: Ask clients to look at Handout 2.5: Missing Links Analysis, and explain how to complete the missing links analysis (MLA) step by step. Emphasize that MLA is a valuable tool for analyzing behavior and goes beyond the factors that led to the problem (BCA). By completing an MLA, clients can identify various factors that hindered them from fulfilling their obligations or working toward their goals.

While clients are working on their MLA, it is important to mention the benefits of this exercise. This will help them not only to understand the specific behavior they are examining, but also to generalize the skills they acquire through skills training. It is highly likely that these clients may exhibit antisocial or problematic behaviors; by using the MLA, they can gain insights into underlying factors that contribute to these behaviors. Make sure you provide clients with feedback and questions that they may not have considered.

After completing the MLA, I ask clients if there was ever a time they used effective self-talk or redirected their behavior to avoid engaging in a problematic behavior. Most clients typically can think of some point in their life where they avoided acting on an impulse or behaving in a problematic manner. Ask them to describe what they did in that instance. Follow up with praise and let them know that they have already used skillful behavior to avoid problem behaviors in the past, and are thus already equipped with some of the tools necessary to make effective choices. I have noticed that many clients feel empowered by this because they tend to enter therapy with low self-regard and self-doubt.

Example of an MLA

Let's use Gio's scenario again. This time we know that Gio tends to flirt with women when he and his wife have problems in their marriage:

- Did Gio know what skillful behavior to use in this situation? Yes. He knew that drinking alcohol had led to him engaging in ineffective and illegal behaviors in the past.
- Was Gio willing to use an effective skill to avoid the behavior? No. Gio told himself that he was going out with his friends to decompress from a stressful week. He further told himself that he was "only" going to have one drink, despite the fact that he has an alcohol addiction.
- What problems got in the way of Gio making wise choices?
  - He did not talk to his wife about their problems or his feelings.
  - He chose to go to the bar with his friends—something that has always been a trigger for him to drink in the past.
  - He told himself that he could only have one drink.
  - He began masturbating to fantasies about Marissa.

Mindfulness and the Stages of Change[12]

Skills Trainer: Many treatment programs utilize the Stages of Change, a transtheoretical model that allows clients to assess their readiness for change. Using this model with your clients can be helpful both to them and to you in terms of understanding where they see themselves in the change process. However, caution is warranted, as the client may see themselves as ahead or behind the empirically derived stage of change according to assessment tools (e.g., VRS-SO[13]).[14]

Ask your client to take out a copy of Handout 2.6: The Stages of Change. Begin the discussion by emphasizing that living life mindfully and effectively tends to lead to individuals accomplishing their goals. To initiate this process, be sure to encourage your client to identify and explain the aspects of his life that he wants to change in order to achieve his goals.

Next, ask the client to share two or three aspects of his life that he wants to change. Some of the responses will include statements such as, "Not going back to prison," "Getting off probation/parole," or "Getting off the sex offender registry" Let them know that they are on the right path, as they have recognized factors within their control. However, guide them to delve deeper and specify the necessary changes they need to implement to avoid reoffending and returning to prison, or to successfully complete probation/parole.

Finally, explain the Stages of Change and how the model can be helpful in terms of understanding where one is in the process of change, where they would like to be, and some preliminary things they will need to do to move to the next stage.

Skills Trainer: Explain each stage.

- **Precontemplation:** When people are in the precontemplation stage, they are not in a place in their lives where they see something as a problem or want to take action. As such, they typically believe that the "cons" outweigh the "pros" when it comes to changing the behavior.
- **Contemplation:** When people are in the contemplation stage, they are considering making a change within six months; however, they are not quite ready to do so yet. People in this stage recognize that their behavior may be unhealthy, unhelpful, or illegal, but remain ambivalent about changing their behavior.
- **Preparation/determination:** In this stage, people are ready to take action within the next month. People in this stage recognize that their behavior is unhealthy, unhelpful, or illegal, and see that

the "pros" of changing the behavior outweigh the "cons." These individuals begin to take small steps to prepare for taking the step into the action stage.

- **Action:** Individuals in this stage have begun to take direct action, and intend to keep moving forward with the behavioral change. These individuals can demonstrate their changes by applying new skills to their lives.
- **Maintenance:** In this stage, people have sustained their behavior change for a while (defined as more than six months), and intend to maintain the behavior change going forward. People in this stage work to prevent relapse to earlier stages.
- **Lapse:** Regardless of the stage they are in (including maintenance), a person may begin to lapse by reverting to old behaviors that led up to their offense. In other words, they begin to use the same thoughts, self-talk, and behaviors that got them into trouble in the first place—for example, lying, procrastinating, not following the rules of their conditions of supervision, denying, minimizing, and justifying one's actions. When an individual is in this stage, they have difficulty moving forward without intervention.

Handout 2.1: Living a Wise Life

This is what a living a wise life looks like to me (be sure to explain):

1. _____
2. _____
3. _____
4. _____
5. _____

Now, list the things you are good at:

1. _____
2. _____
3. _____
4. _____
5. _____

Homework: Goals for living a wise life

Identify four or five goals you have for your life. At least two must be short-term goals. After you have listed the goals, describe what actions you are taking to meet them. If you have not yet begun working toward your goals, describe how you will employ your strengths to meet them.

	Strengths I am using to meet my goal	Things in my environment that are preventing me from meeting my goal	Steps I must take to reach my goal
Goal 1			
Goal 2			
Goal 3			

	Strengths I am using to meet my goal	Things in my environment that are preventing me from meeting my goal	Steps I must take to reach my goal
Goal 4			
Goal 5			
Goal 6			

Handout 2.2: The Feeling Wheel

How do I know whether I am experiencing a primary or secondary emotion?

- **Primary:**
    - Am I experiencing an emotion directly related to a situation or event?
    - Once the event ended, did the emotion go away?
- **Secondary:**
    - Is this emotion becoming more intense?
    - Am I experiencing this emotion beyond the point when the situation/ event has ended?
    - Is the emotion difficult to understand?

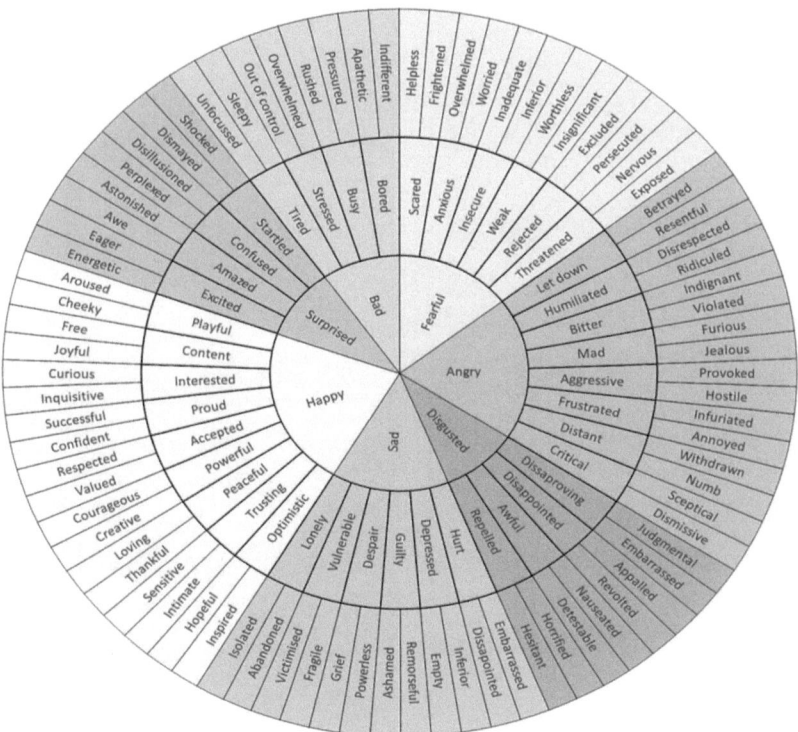

Image 2.1 Feeling Wheel

Handout 2.3: Daily Diary Cards

Abbreviations

- Mast = Masturbate
  Sub = Substance use
- Off = Offend
- Iso = Isolate
- Anx = Anxiety
- Aroused: Refers to sexual fantasies and/or compulsive thoughts

Top Portion

Highest urge to:　　*Strongest emotion each day:*　　*Actions:*

Circle day of Week	Mast	Sub	Off	Anger	Sad	Happy	Anx	Aroused	Mast	Lie	Iso	Lost temper	Off	Skills
Mon														
Tues														
Wed														
Thurs														
Fri														
Sat														
Sun														

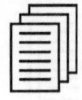

Bottom Portion

Circle the day you practiced each skill

Mindfulness Skills	M	T	W	Th	F	Sat	Sun
Wise Mind							
Observe							
Describe							
Participate							
Nonjudgmental							
One-mindful							
Effective							

Emotion Regulation Skills	M	T	W	Th	F	Sat	Sun
CALM							
CLASP							
Mindful Mast.							
Stopped a fantasy using aversion or other method							

Sexual Regulation Skills	M	T	W	Th	F	Sat	Sun
CALM							
CLASP							
Mindful mast.							
Stopped a fantasy using aversion or other method							

Interpersonal Effectiveness Skills	M	T	W	Th	F	Sa	Sun
CALM							
CLASP							
Mindful mast.							
Stopped a fantasy using aversion or other method							

Distress Tolerance Skills	M	T	W	Th	F	Sat	Sun
Improved the moment							
Radically accepted							
STOP							
COBB							
Self-soothed							
Mindful of current thoughts							

Handout 2.4: Behavior Chain Analysis[15]

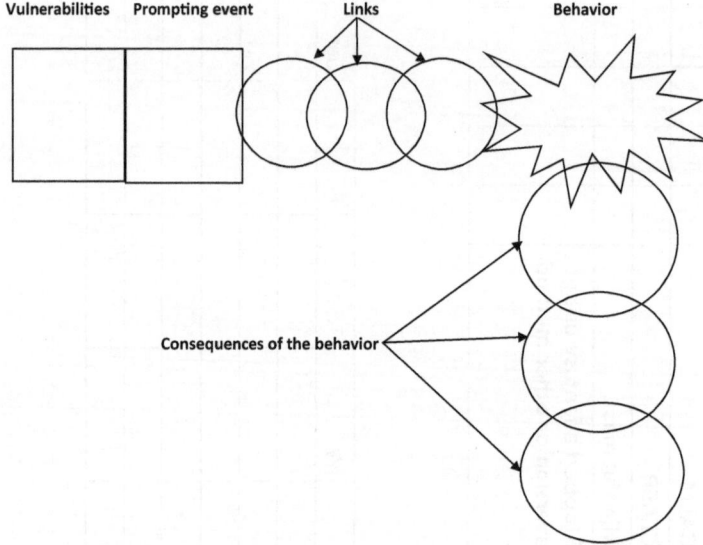

Image 2.2 Behavior Chain Analysis

Steps for completing a behavior chain analysis (BCA):

- Describe the **problem behavior** (rate it on a scale of 1–10, where 1 is the least severe and 10 is the most severe).
- Describe the **prompting event** that started the chain of events leading to the problem behavior.
- Describe the factors happening before the event that made you feel **vulnerable** to starting down the chain of events toward the problem behavior.
- Describe, in detail, the **chain of events** that led to the problem behavior.
- Describe the **consequences** of the problem behavior.

Changing the behavior

- Describe the **skillful behavior** you can use to replace the problem links in the chain of events.
- Develop **prevention plans** to reduce vulnerability to stressful events.
- **Repair** important or significant consequences of the problem behavior

Handout 2.5: Missing Links Analysis (MLA)

Ask yourself the following questions:

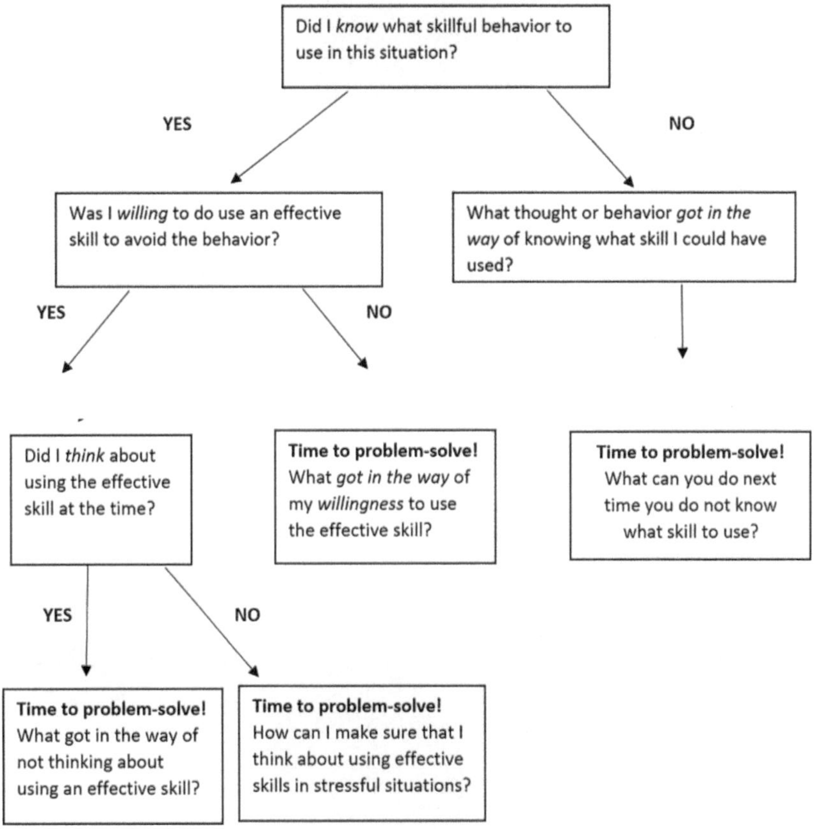

Did I *know* what skillful behavior to use in this situation?

YES → **Was I *willing* to do use an effective skill to avoid the behavior?**

NO → **What thought or behavior *got in the way* of knowing what skill I could have used?**

From "Was I willing...":

YES → **Did I *think* about using the effective skill at the time?**

NO → **Time to problem-solve!** What *got in the way* of my *willingness* to use the effective skill?

From "What thought or behavior got in the way...":

Time to problem-solve! What can you do next time you do not know what skill to use?

From "Did I think about using the effective skill at the time?":

YES → **Time to problem-solve!** What got in the way of not thinking about using an effective skill?

NO → **Time to problem-solve!** How can I make sure that I think about using effective skills in stressful situations?

Handout 2.6: The Stages of Change

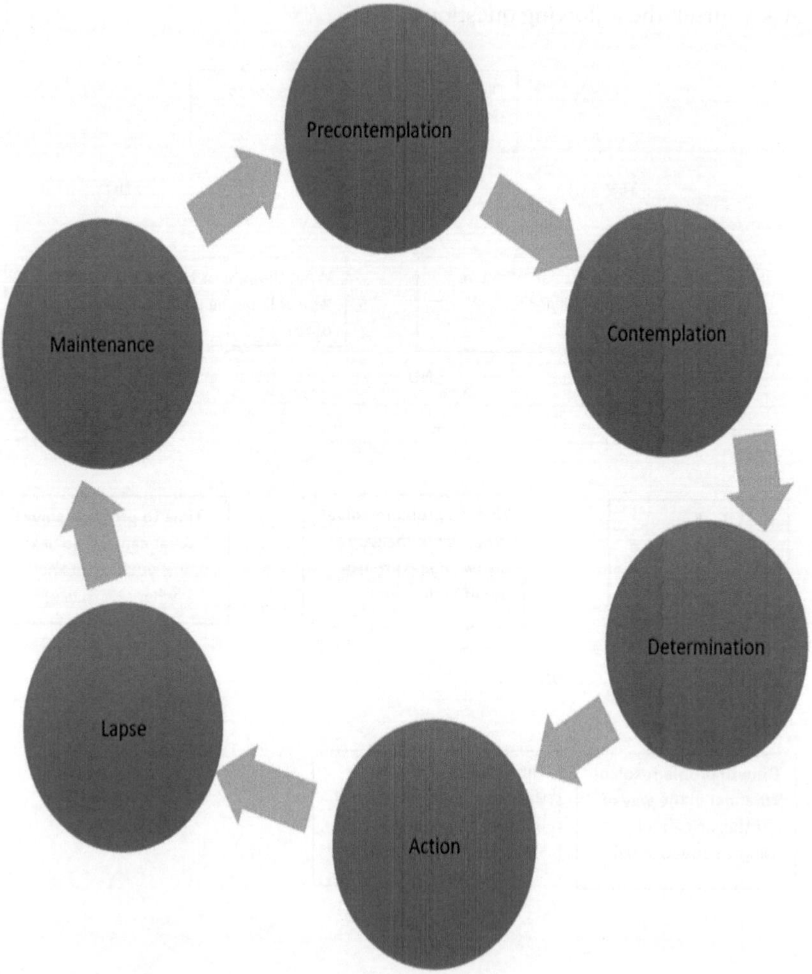

Precontemplation

Contemplation

Determination

Action

Lapse

Maintenance

Image 2.3 Stages of Change

Handout 2.7: Pros and Cons of Practicing Skills

Describe your problem or situation (3–5):

1. _____

   _____

   _____

   _____

2. _____

   _____

   _____

   _____

3. _____

   _____

   _____

   _____

4. _____

   _____

   _____

   _____

5. _____

   _____

   _____

   _____

Describe your goal for each problem or situation:

1. _____
   _____
   _____
   _____

2. _____
   _____
   _____
   _____

3. _____
   _____
   _____
   _____

4. _____
   _____
   _____
   _____

5. _____
   _____
   _____
   _____

Now, make a list of the pros and cons of practicing your skills in each situation:

Pros	Practicing Skills	Not Practicing Skills
	_____	_____
	_____	_____
	_____	_____
	_____	_____
Cons	Practicing Skills	Not Practicing Skills
	_____	_____
	_____	_____
	_____	_____
	_____	_____

Pros	Practicing Skills	Not Practicing Skills
	_____	_____
	_____	_____
	_____	_____
	_____	_____
Cons	Practicing Skills	Not Practicing Skills
	_____	_____
	_____	_____
	_____	_____
	_____	_____

Pros	Practicing Skills	Not Practicing Skills
	_____	_____
	_____	_____
	_____	_____
	_____	_____
Cons	Practicing Skills	Not Practicing Skills
	_____	_____
	_____	_____
	_____	_____
	_____	_____

Pros	Practicing Skills	Not Practicing Skills
	_____ _____ _____ _____	_____ _____ _____ _____
Cons	Practicing Skills	Not Practicing Skills
	_____ _____ _____ _____	_____ _____ _____ _____

Pros	Practicing Skills	Not Practicing Skills
	_____ _____ _____ _____	_____ _____ _____ _____
Cons	Practicing Skills	Not Practicing Skills
	_____ _____ _____ _____	_____ _____ _____ _____

Notes

1　Deci & Ryan (1985).
2　Ward & Gannon (2006).
3　Prescott (2014); Prescott & Wilson (2013).
4　Marshall & Marshall (2014).
5　Harned, Chapman, Dexter-Mazza, Murray, & Comtois (2008).
6　Marshall & Marshall (2014).
7　Mossière & Serin (2015).
8　While attitudes tolerant of sexual offending are related to recidivism (Hanson & Harris, 2000), Hanson & Bussière (1998) and Hanson & Morton-Bourgon (2005) found no relationship between denial of sexual offense and sexual offense recidivism in either treated or untreated offenders in their seminal research.
9　Sakdalan & Gupta (2014). These terms are used interchangeably throughout the book.
10　For further discussion of implementing a strengths-based approach in sex offender treatment, please see de Vries Robbe, Mann, Maruna, & Thornton (2015); Ward & Gannon (2006); and Willis et al. (2020).
11　Linehan (1993; 2015).
12　Modified from Miller and Rollnick (2013). I argue that the term "lapse" is more appropriate than "relapse," because it refers to an event in which the individual is engaging in risky thoughts and behavior that could lead to reoffending (e.g., masturbating to fantasies of children, though not viewing child pornography or offending against a child; see Pithers, 1990; Ward & Hudson, 1996; Ward & Purvis, & Devilly, 2004). "Relapse," on the other hand, refers to a reoffence. This is further discussed in Chapter 17.
13　Violence Risk Scale–Sexual Offense version (VRS-SO; Olver, Wong, Nicholaichuk, & Gordon, 2007).
14　Sakdalan (2023; personal communication).
15　Linehan (1993; 2015).

References

Deci E. L., & Ryan R. M. (1985). The general causality orientations scale: Self-determination in personality. *Journal of Research in Personality, 19*, 109–134. https://doi.org/10.1016/0092-6566(85)90023-6

de Vries Robbe M., Mann R. E., Maruna S. & Thornton D. (2015). An exploration of protective factors supporting desistance from sexual offending. *Sexual Abuse, 27*(1), 16–33. https://doi.org/10.1177/1079063214547582

Hanson R. K., & Bussière M. T. (1998). Predicting relapse: A meta-analysis of sexual offender recidivism studies. *Journal of Consulting and Clinical Psychology, 66*(2), 348–362. https://doi.org/10.1037/0022-006X.66.2.348

Hanson R. K., & Harris A. J. R. (2000). Where should we intervene? Dynamic predictors of sexual assault recidivism. *Criminal Justice and Behavior*, 27(1), 6–35. https://doi.org/10.1177/0093854800027001002

Hanson R. K., & Morton-Bourgon K. E. (2005). The characteristics of persistent sexual offenders: A meta-analysis of recidivism studies. *Journal of Consulting and Clinical Psychology*, 73(6), 1154–1163. https://doi.org/10.1037/0022-006X.73.6.1154

Harned M. S., Chapman A. L., Dexter-Mazza E. T., Murray A., & Comtois K. A. (2008). Enhancing attachment security in the treatment of borderline personality disorder. *Journal of Consulting and Clinical Psychology*, 76(4), 756–766. https://doi.org/10.1037/0022-006X.76.4.756

Linehan M. M (1993). Cognitive-Behavioral Treatment of Borderline Personality Disorder. New York: Guilford Publications.

Linehan M. M. (2015). *Skills Training Manual* (2nd ed.). New York: Guilford Press.

Marshall W. L., & Marshall L. E. (2014). Therapeutic process. In Carich M. S., & Mussack S. E. (eds.). *The Safer Society Handbook of Sexual Abuser Assessment and Treatment*. Brandon, VT. The Safer Society Press.

Miller W. R., & Rollnick S. (2013). *Motivational Interviewing: Helping People Change*. (3rd edition). New York: Guilford Press.

Mossière A., & Serin R. C. (2015). A critique of models and measures of treatment readiness in offenders. *Aggression and Violent Behavior*, 22, 71–82. https://doi.org/10.1016/j.avb.2015.03.004

Olver M. E., Wong S. C., Nicholaichuk T., & Gordon A. (2007). The validity and reliability of the Violence Risk Scale-Sexual Offender version: Assessing sex offender risk and evaluating therapeutic change. *Psychological Assessment*, 19(3), 318–329. https://doi.org/10.1037/1040-3590.19.3.318

Pithers W. D. (1990). Relapse prevention with sexual aggressors. In: Marshall W. L., Laws D. R., Barbaree H. E. (eds) *Handbook of Sexual Assault*. Boston, MA: Springer.

Prescott D. P., & Wilson R. J. (2013). *Awakening Motivation for Difficult Changes*. Holyoke, MA: NEARI Press.

Prescott D. P. (2014) Therapeutic process. In Carich M. S., & Mussack S. E. (eds.). *The Safer Society Handbook of Sexual Abuser Assessment and Treatment*. Brandon, VT: The Safer Society Press.

Sakdalan J. A., & Gupta R. (2014). Wise mind—risky mind: A reconceptualisation of dialectical behaviour therapy concepts and its application to sexual offender treatment. *Journal of Sexual Aggression*, 20(1), 110–120. https://doi.org/10.1080/13552600.2012.724457

Ward T., & Gannon T. A. (2006). Rehabilitation, etiology, and self-regulation: The comprehensive good lives model of treatment for sexual offenders. *Aggression and Violent Behavior*, 11(1), 77–94. https://doi.org/10.1016/j.avb.2005.06.001

Willis G. M., Kelley S. M., & Thornton D. (2020). Are protective factors valid constructs? Interrater reliability and construct validity of proposed protective factors against sexual reoffending. *Criminal Justice and Behavior*, 47(11), 1448–1467. https://doi.org/10.1177/0093854820941039

Group Dynamics and Expectations, and the Biopsychosocial Model of Sexual Offending

3

Skills Trainer: In the skills trainer role, it is essential to create and reinforce a positive and engaging atmosphere. Begin your first group session by introducing yourself and then encourage group members to introduce themselves as well. To foster a sense of positivity and connection, ask each group member to share something positive that has occurred in their lives during the past week. This activity sets a welcoming tone, promotes engagement, and allows group members to start their treatment group on a positive note.

To create a safe environment, it is important to establish ground rules for both group members and skills trainers. Engage the group in a discussion about what they need from one another and from the skills trainers to feel comfortable in the treatment group, and write down agreed-upon rules on a large sheet of paper or whiteboard. Ensure, once again, that confidentiality is addressed and understood, and clarify what it includes and does not include. Be sure to emphasize that clients should not have contact with one another outside of the group setting due to probation/parole conditions, to reduce the likelihood of collusion between group members, and to reduce the likelihood of therapy-interfering behaviors. If participants come to a group under the influence of drugs or alcohol, they will be asked to leave. The incident will be discussed with the client's individual therapist, who will help the client complete a behavior chain analysis to address the behavior.

DOI: 10.4324/9781003451099-5

The Biopsychosocial Model

One goal of research is to gain a deeper understanding of the biological, psychological, and social factors that contribute to sex offending. Similar to Linehan's (1993) incorporation of the biosocial model in treatment with women with borderline personality disorder, the skills trainer will address the various biological, psychological, and social components of sexual offending with clients. Be sure to "keep it simple" by discussing the information presented in the following section.

Factors Involved in Sexual Offending: A Biosocial Model

Biological psychologists and criminologists have found various etiological factors that contribute to adverse childhood experiences (ACEs), and a greater likelihood of engaging in sexually abusive behavior. [1]

In 2013, the Centers for Disease Control and Prevention released its landmark study which revealed the impact of ACEs on individuals' future health and mental health outcomes, and behavior.[2] The study addressed two domains: household dysfunction (e.g., parent separation, parental substance abuse and mental health problems, and parental incarceration), and childhood maltreatment (e.g., emotional, physical, and sexual abuse; emotional and physical neglect). Specifically, the research demonstrated that the more ACEs an individual experienced in childhood, the greater the likelihood of that individual experiencing mental health problems, chronic stress, trouble regulating their emotions, and ultimately behavioral problems.

A threshold score of four ACEs is indicative of increased vulnerability to unfavorable outcomes. An increase in ACEs creates a cumulative and multiplicative effect on the individual, [3] which can alter brain development and plasticity, and lead to behavioral problems.[4] When people are confronted with a perceived threat, they experience a "fight-or-flight" response. This response is driven by the body's increased production of the hormones adrenaline and cortisol. Once the perceived threat has ceased, most people's body returns to baseline, and they experience a decrease in adrenaline and cortisol levels. However, some people are more prone to stressors than others, either because of genetics or due to their environment.[5]

In fact, research has shown that the cumulative effect of stress negatively impacts parts of the brain—particularly the limbic system[6]—leading to problems such as an overactive amygdala, which can cause hyperarousal, an increased fear response, and emotional disorders and dysregulation.[7] On the other hand, it can also lead to an underactive amygdala and a reduction in cortical activity, which are associated with antisocial personality disorder and psychopathy traits.[8] In a 2016 study, researchers found a link between ACE scores—specifically physical abuse in childhood—and psychopathic personality traits, and externalizing behavior.[9] Higher ACE scores are associated with higher-risk sex offender populations.[10] Moreover, research has consistently shown that individuals who have committed sexual offenses have higher ACE scores than offenders who have not committed sexual offenses,[11] and the general population.[12] Of note, sexual offenders are significantly more likely than non-sexual offenders to have specifically experienced sexual abuse in childhood.[13] As such, understanding clients' individual ACEs can assist clinicians in identifying client vulnerabilities such as fear of relationships because they may result in abandonment, mistrust, and emotional deprivation.

When stressors are constantly present, an individual's hormone levels do not return to baseline, and overexposure to these hormones leads to various negative health and mental health outcomes.[14] If a mother experiences high levels of stress throughout her life, or pregnancy, she is at increased likelihood of passing along genetic problems to her child, as chronic stress and trauma lead to changes in gene expression in the brain.[15] Additionally, mothers who experience chronic stress or trauma may find it more difficult to form a healthy attachment with their children.[16] Consistent, loving responses to their infants' needs typically lay the groundwork for a secure, organized parent-child relationship, and an individual's likelihood to have secure interpersonal relationships.[17]

For example, children who experience an insecure attachment with their primary caregiver are more likely than children with a secure attachment to face challenges forming healthy and secure emotional connections with others, including intimate relationships.[18] This lack of secure attachment can lead to a range of psychological and interpersonal challenges, such as low self-esteem, poor coping skills, and inadequate interpersonal skills.[19] Difficulties in these areas can make it challenging for these individuals to establish healthy emotional connections and navigate appropriate boundaries in relationships.[20] As a result, they may struggle to develop intimate relationships characterized by trust, empathy, and mutual respect; and they are more likely to interact with others in an aggressive/hostile manner, use sex as a coping mechanism, and develop emotional congruence with children.[21] Finally, exposure to adverse life experiences also leads to high-risk behaviors such as early onset of sexual activity, a high number of sexual partners, hypersexuality, and substance abuse.

In sum, higher ACE scores are associated with higher rates of offending in general, and specifically among men who have committed sexual offenses. These individuals are also more likely to experience more ACEs, thus producing a cumulative effect and increasing the likelihood of engaging in maladaptive behaviors in adulthood. Individuals who experience family dysfunction and maltreatment in childhood are more likely than those who have not experienced these problems to form a secure attachment to their primary caregiver(s), and may experience a sense of emotional emptiness or loneliness, seeking alternative and maladaptive ways to fulfill their unmet emotional needs. In some cases, this may lead to seeking sexual gratification as a means of compensating for the perceived emotional deficit. The lack of secure attachment during childhood may contribute to a distorted understanding of intimacy, leading to the sexualization of relationships and an inability to distinguish appropriate boundaries.[22]

> **Skills Trainer:** Explain that most people do not wake up one morning and say, "Hey, I think I'll commit a sexual offense today." In fact, when asked how they planned their offense, why they offended, or what they were thinking during the offense, offenders usually say, "I don't know. I just wasn't thinking."
>
> One of the goals of treatment is to help the client synthesize the dialectic of knowing that they did something that violated the law, the conditions of probation or incarceration, and the personal boundaries of others—even if they are still unable to admit to their sexual offense(s)—and not knowing why they did it.

We know that certain biological factors are associated with a higher likelihood of future offending. For example, if a pregnant woman uses alcohol, drugs, or cigarettes, or does not get the nutrition she needs during pregnancy, the baby's brain development can be affected. Further, the baby can be affected if the mother experiences frequent stressors during her pregnancy or post-partum, such as abuse, homelessness, or chronic health problems. But why might these

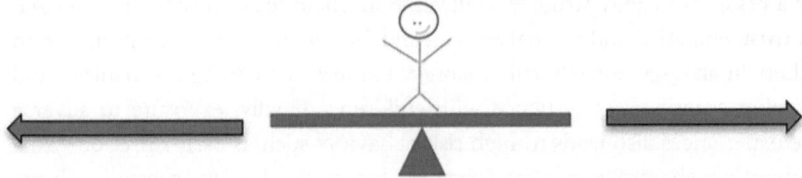

Image 3.1 Balance

factors harm the child? When an individual faces a real or perceived threat, they experience a "fight-or-flight" response. This response happens because your body releases extra hormones to help you get through a stressful situation. But once the threat goes away, most people's bodies return to baseline, or "normal." This means that the fight-or-flight hormones decrease. However, some people have more stressors in their lives than others, either because of genetics or due to their environment. When stressors are constantly present, a person's hormone levels do not return to baseline, and over time these hormones lead to negative health and mental health outcomes (see mayoclinic.org), such as:

- Addiction.
- Anger.
- Anxiety.
- Depression.
- Digestive problems.
- Headaches.
- Muscle tension and pain.
- Heart disease.
- High blood pressure and stroke.
- Memory and concentration impairment.
- Obesity.
- Sleep problems.

Some of these symptoms—such as addiction, anger, anxiety, and depression—have been linked to offending.

Some children witness or experience ongoing negative, unhealthy situations in their lives that cause trauma. We call these "adverse childhood experiences," or "ACEs." These can include, but are not limited to, the following factors:

- Physically or emotionally absent parents.
- Abuse/violence in the home.
- Growing up in a dangerous/violent neighborhood.
- Parents who abuse drugs or alcohol.

Overall, unhealthy social circumstances or environments may, in part, have a negative impact on an individual's life outlook, relationships, and unhealthy thoughts and behaviors. When a person is frequently exposed to these kinds of situations, they are at a higher risk of other life problems, such as a negative or unhealthy view of themselves and others, poor coping skills, poor decision making, and illegal or risky behaviors.

Children who grow up in a negative, unhealthy environment are more likely than children who grow up in a happy, stable environment to participate in high-risk behaviors such as having first-time intercourse at a young age; having a lot of sexual partners; being overly sexual in circumstances where it is not appropriate; and substance abuse.

Let's take a look at an example of an individual with high-risk behaviors: John has always been attracted to children. He knows it is illegal to have sexual contact with children, so instead he decides to place himself in situations where children will be present. He joins a local church and volunteers to teach youth Sunday school, and volunteers to coach peewee football, all so he can be closer to children. After volunteering, John goes home, fantasizes about the children, and masturbates until he has an orgasm. John's behavior is high risk because he has increased his exposure to children. Increased exposure can lead to increased desire to offend against a child. In addition, because he is in a position of trust, he may more readily be able to groom a child and position himself so that he is alone with a child. After masturbating to fantasies about the children, John feels bad and drinks alcohol until he numbs his feelings.

Finally, the quality of attachment between parent and infant plays a crucial role in child development, and the ability to be effective in one's interpersonal relationships. "Attachment" refers to the emotional bond between an infant and their primary caregiver, usually their parents. When the caregiver is sensitive and attentive to a baby's needs—such as feeding the baby when they are hungry, changing diapers when soiled, and soothing the baby when they are upset—this impacts infants' anticipation of caregivers' response to their needs. This awareness can develop as early as six months old.[23] There are four types of attachment a child may develop toward their caregiver:

- ***Secure:** Secure attachment is considered an organized strategy that a baby develops to cope with distress because the baby learns that the parent will address their various needs when they arise.*
- ***Insecure-avoidant:** Insecure-avoidant attachment occurs when the caregiver responds negatively to the infant's distress (e.g., by getting annoyed, or ignoring it). The infant learns their needs will not be met by the caregiver, and thus learns to avoid the caregiver when they experience distress. Insecure-avoidant attachment has been shown to lead to adjustment problems, inflexibility, and overcompensation by only relying on oneself later in life.*
- ***Insecure-ambivalent:** Insecure-ambivalent attachment occurs when the caregiver responds inconsistently to the baby's distress. The child does not learn which behaviors will elicit which type of response, and thus*

behaves inconsistently with others. Insecure-ambivalent attachment has been found to lead to increased emotional dysregulation, and risk of social problems.

- ***Insecure-disorganized:*** *This type of attachment is formed when a caregiver neglects or is abusive toward the infant. The child is raised in an invalidating environment, and thus learns to distrust others and their intentions.*

Let's look at an example of an individual who has experienced insecure attachment with his parents: Trevor was 22 years old when he entered prison on a sexual assault charge. His mother left the family when he was three, and he was raised by an abusive, controlling, alcoholic father. Trevor never felt close to his father because he was afraid of him. He had no other positive role models to guide him through healthy, normative development. Trevor, by his own admission, was an awkward child, had poor social skills, and was picked on by other kids. He eventually started hanging out with other boys who also had limited social skills (i.e., they were immature). At age 20, Trevor met Katie, age 13, and felt a connection with her. He believed they had much in common, and that they had an intimate connection. They ended up having a sexual relationship. Trevor was charged with sexual assault of a minor, as Katie's age rendered her unable to legally consent to sex.

Notes

1 Men who engage in sexually deviant behavior exhibit various motivational and facilitating factors for offending (Seto 2008, 2019). The Motivation-Facilitation Model of sexual offending draws upon previous theoretical models of criminality (e.g., Finkelhor, 1984; Gottfredson & Hirschi, 1990) and empirically explains how dysfunction within the sexual domain (e.g., paraphilias, high sex drive, and intense mating effort) is a motivating factor for sexual offending; whereas factors related to antisociality (e.g., problems with self-regulation, hostility toward women, negative affect, and substance use) facilitate sexual offending.

2 Centers for Disease Control and Prevention (2013a, 2013b).

3 Putnam, Harris, & Putnam (2013).

4 Kahn, Jackson, Keiser, Ambroziak, & Levenson (2021).

5 McEwen (2016).

6 The limbic system is made up of various structures in the brain that aid in emotional processing and regulation, organization of goals, and physiological responses, and is responsible for long-term memory which modifies emotions.

7 Grant, Cannistraci, Hollon, Gore, & Shelton (2011).
8 Birbaumer, Veit, Lotze, Erb, Hermann, Grodd, & Flor (2005).
9 Dargis, Newman, & Koenigs (2016).
10 Kahn et al. (2021).
11 Revis, Looman, Franco, & Rojas (2013).
12 Levenson et al. (2016).
13 For example, Reavis, Looman, Franco, and Rojas (2013) found that sexual offenders report higher scores on the ACE scale—specifically related to physical, emotional, and sexual abuse—than the general population. Additionally, studies show that approximately 26% to 38% of all sexual offenders have a history of being sexually abused (Levenson, Willis, & Prescott, 2016); and that sexual offenders are more than three times as likely to experience sexual abuse than non-sexual offenders (Jespersen, Lalumiere, & Seto, 2009).
14 Dziurkowska & Wesolowski (2021).
15 McEwen (2016).
16 Ainsworth, Belhar, Waters, & Wall (1978); Anis, Ross, Ntanda, Hart, & Letourneau (2022).
17 Ainsworth et al. (1978).
18 Grady, Levenson, & Bolder (2017).
19 Benoit (2004); Grady et al. (2017).
20 Grady et al. (2017).
21 Beech & Mitchell (2016); Kahn et al. (2021).
22 Grady et al. (2017).
23 Benoit (2004).

References

Anis L., Ross K., Ntanda H., Hart M., & Letourneau N. (2022). Effect of attachment and child health (ATTACHTM) parenting program on parent-infant attachment, parental reflective function, and parental depression. *International Journal of Environmental Research and Public Health, 19*(14), 8425. https://doi.org/10.3390/ijerph19148425

Ainsworth M. D., Belhar M. Waters E., & Wall S. (1978). *Patterns of Attachment.* Hillsdale, NJ: Erlbaum.

Beech A., & Mitchell I. (2016). Intimacy deficits/attachment problems in sexual offenders: Towards a neurobiological explanation. In Boer D. P. (ed.), *The Wiley Blackwell Handbook on Assessment, Treatment and Theories of Sexual Offending*, Volume 1 (Vol. 1). Hoboken, NJ: Wiley.

Benoit D. (2004). Infant-parent attachment: Definition, types, antecedents, measurement and outcome. *Paediatrics & Child Health, 9*(8), 541–545. https://doi.org/10.1093/pch/9.8.541

Birbaumer N., Veit R., Lotze M., Erb M., Hermann C., Grodd W., & Flor H. (2005). Deficientfearconditioninginpsychopathy:Afunctionalmagneticresonanceimaging study. *Archives of General Psychiatry, 62*(7), 799–805. https://doi.org/10.1001/archpsyc.62.7.799

Centers for Disease Control and Prevention. (2013a). Adverse Childhood Experience Study: Major findings. Retrieved from http://www.cdc.gov/ace/findings.htm

Centers for Disease Control and Prevention. (2013b). *Adverse Childhood Experience Study: Risk and Protective Factors.* https://www.cdc.gov/violenceprevention/aces/riskprotectivefactors.html

Dargis M., Newman J., & Koenigs M. (2016). Clarifying the link between childhood abuse History and psychopathic traits in adult criminal offenders. *Personality Disorders, 7*(3), 221–228. https://doi.org/10.1037/per0000147

Dziurkowska E., & Wesolowski M. (2021). Cortisol as a biomarker of mental disorder severity. *Journal of Clinical Medicine, 10*(21), 5204. https://doi.org/10.3390/jcm10215204

Finkelhor D. (1984). *Child Sexual Abuse. New Theory and Research.* New York: Free Press.

Gottfredson M. R., & Hirschi T. (1990). *A General Theory of Crime.* Stanford, CA: Stanford University Press.

Grady M. D., Levenson J. S., & Bolder T. (2017). Linking adverse childhood effects and attachment: A theory of etiology for sexual offending. *Trauma, Violence, & Abuse, 18*(4), 433–444. https://doi.org/10.1177/1524838015627147

Grant M. M., Cannistraci C., Hollon S. D., Gore J., & Shelton R. (2011). Childhood trauma history differentiates amygdala response to sad faces within MDD. *Journal of Psychiatric Research, 45*(7), 886–895. https://doi.org/10.1016/j.jpsychires.2010.12.004

Jespersen A. F., Lalumière M. L., & Seto M. C. (2009). Sexual abuse history among adult sex offenders and non-sex offenders: A meta-analysis. *Child Abuse & Neglect, 33*(3), 179–192. https://doi.org/10.1016/j.chiabu.2008.07.004

Kahn R. E., Jackson K., Keiser K., Ambroziak G., & Levenson J. S. (2021). Adverse childhood experiencing among sexual offenders: Associations with sexual recidivism risk and psychopathology. *Sexual Abuse, 33*(7), 839–866. https://doi.org/10.1177/1079063220970031

Levenson J. S., Willis G. M., & Prescott D. S. (2016). Adverse childhood experiences in the lives of male sex offenders: Implications for trauma-informed care. *Sexual Abuse, 28*(4), 340–359. https://doi.org/10.1177/1079063214535819

McEwen B. S. (2016), In pursuit of resilience: Stress, epigenetics, and brain plasticity. *Annals of the New York Academy of Sciences, 1373*(1), 56–64. https://doi.org/10.1111/nyas.13020

Putnam K. T., Harris W. W., & Putnam F. W. (2013). Synergistic childhood adversities and complex adult psychopathology. *Journal of Traumatic Stress, 26*(4), 435–442. https://doi.org/10.1002/jts.21833

Reavis J. A., Looman J., Franco K. A., & Rojas B. (2013). Adverse childhood experiences and adult criminality: How long must we live before we possess our own lives? *The Permanente Journal, 17*(2), 44–48. https://doi.org/10.7812/TPP/12-072

Seto M. C. (2019). The Motivation-Facilitation Model of sexual offending. *Sexual Abuse, 31*(1), 3–24. https://doi.org/10.1177/1079063217720919

Seto M. C. (2008). *Pedophilia and Sexual Offending against Children: Theory, Assessment, and Intervention.* Washington, DC: American Psychological Association.

Core Mindfulness Skills

4

A Dialectical Approach

Begin by asking clients what a balanced, or "more balanced" life looks like. (I use "balance" rather than "dialectics" for brevity.) How do they know when they are living a balanced life? You will probably notice that your clients perceive balance as "when life is going well for me." Remind them that balance does not necessarily mean life is "good," as we can enjoy our lives when things are out of balance. For example, clients may have really enjoyed and felt good viewing child sexual exploitation material (CSEM) and masturbating to it. Perhaps they feel happy when they drink or use drugs. These activities might be the highlight of their day; however, they do not equate to balance.

You may want to use the example of a seesaw to explain balance.

Ask participants to take out Handout 4.1: Wise Mind/Risky Mind. Their homework is to complete the "homework" section of this handout.

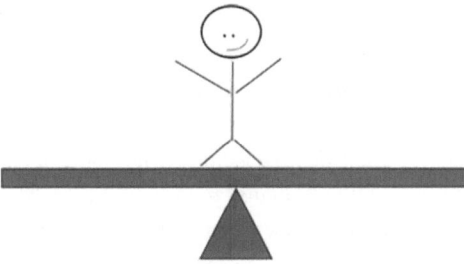

Image 4.1 Balance

DOI: 10.4324/9781003451099-6

Skills Trainer:

"Balance" refers to one's ability to maintain a life that feels at least somewhat stable. In other words, it allows you to navigate your life in such a way that you avoid "falling"—or that you are at least able to "bounce back" after falling. But balance in our lives requires us to practice training our thoughts, feelings, and associated behaviors. There are many people who tend to use "black-and-white" thinking. This type of thinking can be problematic, especially when you frequently react to a situation in an overly emotional manner ("emotional mind"). If you have ever been called "hot-headed," "aggressive," "stubborn," or "difficult to get along with," or have been told that you have a tendency to overreact, you may tend to overuse your emotional mind. This means that you are more likely to react, rather than respond effectively, to an event—for example, by staying in bed for days at a time, yelling, name-calling, hitting, or other unhelpful behavior.

On the other hand, black-and-white thinking can be equally problematic if you completely avoid your emotions and use only the analytic part of your brain, which tends to rationalize things ("reason mind"). While this might sound better than being in emotional mind, the problem is that you may overintellectualize situations that require emotion or empathy. For example, has anyone ever told you that you are "absent," "aloof," or "unemotional"; or that you "just can't relate to others"? If so, this could mean that you tend to overuse your reason mind.

Finally, some of your thoughts, emotions, and choices prior to the sexual offense were very risky and led to the offense. We refer to this as "risky mind."[1] Risky mind overlaps with emotional mind and reason mind. As you can see from Handout 4.1: Wise Mind/Risky Mind, there are elements of risk related to both reason mind and emotional mind.

Notice that overusing emotional mind or reason mind in any given circumstance also leads to risky mind. Staying in one mindset can pose problems in your interpersonal life because your behavior pushes people away—perhaps because they are afraid of you, or emotionally drained by your frequent moodiness or constant problems. Emotional mind is also one way that people get in trouble with the law. For example, you have probably heard men say something like, "She was making out with me, but when I took her clothes off, she told me she didn't want to have sex. How dare she push me away. She was giving me all the signals that she wanted to have sex, so I had sex with her."

Overusing reason mind can also push people away because you are unable to express emotion or empathize with the emotions of others. It can also get you into trouble—especially when you ignore, rationalize, or minimize harmful behavior. For example, men who have used CSEM tend to rationalize their behavior by telling themselves that the children in the images look like they are enjoying themselves, or that they are only viewing images and not physically touching a child. While the children in the images may smile or laugh, and while the viewer is not actually touching a child, they are actively engaging in child exploitation.

How do we find a balance between emotional and reason mind in order to avoid risky mind? Let's take a look at wise mind in order to understand how we can blend emotional and reason minds. When people use their wise mind, they integrate logic and emotion, and can focus on the present. In order to achieve wise mind, mindfulness skills are necessary. Mindfulness draws upon Eastern philosophy and Western medicine, and has demonstrated positive results for a wide range of physical, social, and psychological problems. When an individual can achieve awareness of the present moment, and acknowledge and accept their thoughts, feelings, and physical sensations without fighting them, they are being mindful. In other words, they are fully present in, and conscious of, the moment; and of the connection between their responses to their environment.

Using wise mind can feel challenging at first; however, like any skill we want to improve, mindfulness skills require ongoing practice.

Rewiring Your Brain with Mindfulness

Skills Trainer:
Using the wise mind model is the first step to understanding how you tend to think about, and react to, various situations in your life. Hopefully, this model will serve as a foundation for you to understand what a more balanced and effective life would look like for you, so you can achieve a wise life.

Interestingly, our brains have a unique property called "neuroplasticity." This is the idea that our brains can change and adapt throughout our lives. Brains are flexible and moldable, and we have the power to change their structure and function depending on the activities in which we choose to participate—just like how our muscles can become stronger with exercise, or weaker without exercise. For example, one way in which people change the structure and function of their brains can be through drugs or alcohol. While using substances may make someone feel good in the moment, it has long-term consequences that ultimately make people feel worse than they did before they began using substances. Other ways to change the structure and function of your brain are through exercise, meditation, good nutrition, and making an effort to notice "the good things" in life. As strange as that may sound, research has shown that people who *intentionally look for positive experiences, or see the positive even in negative circumstances, tend to be more content with their lives.[2]*

Mindfulness is a practice that involves being fully present and engaged in the present moment, free from distraction or judgment. It requires us to pay attention to our thoughts, emotions, and sensations as they arise, in order to achieve a heightened state of awareness about what is going on inside our bodies, and around us. As humans, we often get caught up in negative thinking patterns, or become preoccupied with worries and stress, which can cause us to overlook or downplay positive aspects in our lives. By regularly practicing mindfulness, people can stay in their wise mind. Further, it helps them focus on positive moments and experiences, which makes them feel happier and stronger when facing tough times. Mindfulness is like a tool that allows people to appreciate and understand the good things around them. It often helps them feel better and live a more meaningful and fulfilling life. Being mindful requires two sets of skills: what *skills (observe, describe, participate), and* how *skills.*

Note: I encourage my clients to write a positive experience on a slip of paper each day and put it in a large envelope I provide them. They can review these positive experiences when they are "in a rut," or simply want to remember past pleasant experiences.

What and How Skills

Skills Trainer: Ask participants to take out Handout 4.2: Mindfulness Skills: What and How?, and Handout 4.3: A Balanced Approach.

What *skills include observing what is happening both around you and internally, describing what we notice, and participating in the moment. For example, learning to ride a bike is a skill that takes practice. When you first start learning to ride a bike, you have to observe the various parts of the bike that you will use. You observe what it feels like to sit on the seat and stabilize yourself. You adjust yourself to distribute your body weight evenly, so you don't fall. And finally, you begin to pedal. As you are observing your actions—in this case, riding your bike—you also describe what sensations you feel. You might feel nervous about how fast to pedal, or about falling; but the more you participate through practicing—despite falling or pedaling too fast—the more proficient you become. In other words, you can participate in the activity by observing and describing "what works" in order to ride a bike.*

How *skills refer to how we observe, describe, and participate within our environment. In order to effectively observe, describe, and participate to improve our skills, we must do so without judgment or blame. As such, the three* how *skills are: non-judgmental, one-mindful, and effective. Using our* what *skills in a non-judgmental manner means that we avoid attaching an evaluative label to our experiences, ourselves, or others. Instead, the focus stays on consideration of outcomes, or consequences. There are consequences for every behavior— some positive, some negative. A non-judgmental approach encourages us to think about the possible consequences of our behavior and adjust it accordingly. For example, when you learn to ride a bike, you will likely fall off at first. You fall because riding a bike is something new, and you have to figure out what to do to avoid falling. Falling off does not mean you are a "failure," or "stupid"; or that you will never learn how to ride a bike. It simply means you need to continue to practice the skill.*

When attending to ourselves and our environments one-mindfully, we are completely engaged in the moment. That is, we are focused on the moment; not on multitasking or attending to other thoughts that pop into our heads. This is an awareness that some have described as "falling awake."[3] Learning to ride a bike requires significant focus. You probably avoided texting others or viewing your social media as you were learning to ride a bike; had you been focusing on your phone, it would have been virtually impossible to be engaged in your practice. This is because we only have a limited working memory, which means that multitasking is not an effective strategy. If you were completely participating in learning to ride a bike, you were doing so one-mindfully.

The final how *skill has to do with how effectively you observe, describe, and participate. Being effective means that you do not dwell on immediate gratification, or "being right," or immediately becoming proficient at the skill, but rather focus on doing what needs to be done to reach your goal. If, for example, you know how to ride a bike, you know that it takes time to learn the skill. Expecting to ride perfectly the first, second, or third time is unrealistic and sets people up for failure. Therefore, effectively managing our expectations allows us to be mindful of our environments, actions, and physiological responses.*

Ask participants to take out Handout 4.4: FLOURISH Skills for Living a Wise Life and review it with them.

I typically begin the initial four or five groups by engaging in a mindfulness exercise aimed at honing clients' *what* and *how* skills. I encourage clients to begin their practice by identifying and articulating solely what they observe through their senses, and excluding thoughts and emotions. It is noteworthy that certain clients—particularly those that display narcissistic traits or frequently succumb to emotion-driven thinking—may encounter difficulties with these exercises. This challenge arises from their tendency to fixate on their own thoughts and emotions, often perceiving them as incontrovertible truths. Your role, then, is to facilitate your clients' journey toward accepting things at face value before interjecting emotions or acting upon their interpretations. The following is a compilation of activities that I use with clients to cultivate the fundamental aspects of observation and description using their senses:

- Environment: Ask clients to turn their attention to where they are and what they are doing in the moment. For example, encourage them to look around the room and quietly identify sensations in their bodies, and what they see, hear, and smell. I usually give clients one minute to observe, describe, and fully participate, and then go around the room and ask them to share a few things they noticed.
- Sensations: Allow clients one or two minutes to observe their bodily sensations in the moment. Ask them what they noticed and how they felt being fully present in the moment.
- Objects: Give each client an object, such as a shell or stone. Allow them one or two minutes to fully engage with it and describe how it looks and what it feels like, without attaching emotions or labels. Go around the room and ask clients what they noticed.
- Food: Give clients a taste of three different food items. For example, I typically give clients a small plate with a cracker, a strawberry, and a gummy bear, and ask them to use their senses to describe each item without labeling it. Some clients will say that something tastes "nasty" or "good." Gently remind them to avoid using labels and stick to describing only what they see, feel, smell, or taste.
- Music: This can be tricky, and I usually reserve this for the final *what/how* skills exercise. Choose three songs from different genres. Play each song for one minute and ask clients to jot down words that reflect *only* what they hear. Music tends to elicit feelings, thoughts, and memories of experiences, so you will notice that clients may struggle to focus solely on what they hear. Once you have completed the exercise, ask clients to choose one of the songs to describe. In my experience, most clients do not include lyrics on their list, which elicits a discussion about hearing what others say.

Once the group has become acquainted with the essential *what/how* skills, I begin every group session by engaging in a weekly mindfulness meditation exercise. Initially, we embark on a two-minute mindfulness practice, gradually increasing it by an additional minute each week until we reach a duration of 10 minutes. Once clients have worked their way up to the 10-minute mark, we remain at 10-minute mindfulness practices before beginning each group. For a comprehensive list of ideas, please refer to Handout 16.2: CABB Skills.

Handout 4.1: Wise Mind/Risky Mind[4]

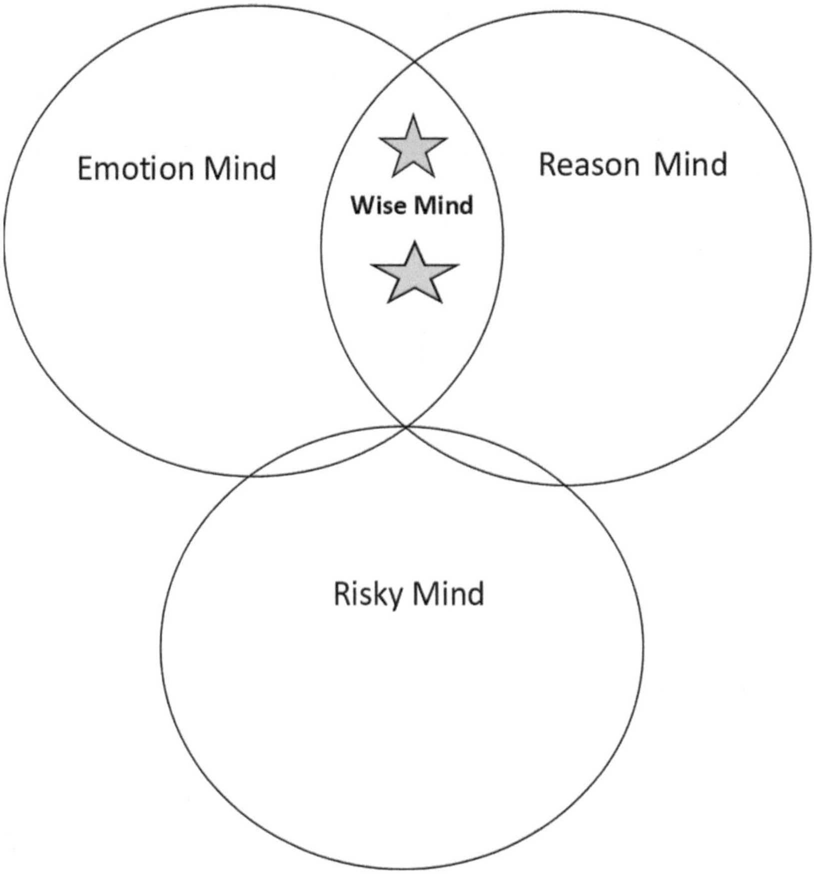

Emotion Mind

Reason Mind

Wise Mind

Risky Mind

Image 4.2 Wise Mind- Risky Mind

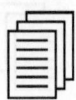

Homework: Reason mind, emotional mind, risky mind, and wise mind

When I am in reason mind, my thoughts, feelings, and behaviors look like this (e.g., "I resort to overthinking"; "I push my feelings away"; "I ignore the situation"):

_____

_____

_____

_____

_____

_____

_____

When I am in emotional mind, my thoughts, feelings, and behaviors look like this (e.g., "I think the other person is stupid"; "I feel angry"; "I lash out and yell at the other person"):

_____

_____

_____

_____

_____

_____

_____

_____

When I am in risky mind, my thoughts, feelings, and behaviors look like this (e.g., "I think about viewing child sexual exploitation material"; "I feel anxious"; "I view adult pornography"):

_____

_____

_____

_____

_____

_____

_____

_____

When I am in wise mind, my thoughts, feelings, and behaviors look like this (e.g., "I think about my response before acting"; "I feel calm/anxious/ frustrated"; "I tell the other person I need to think about the situation for a few minutes before responding"):

_____

_____

_____

_____

_____

_____

_____

_____

Handout 4.2: Mindfulness Skills: *What* and *How*

What skills

What skills help you to be present and engage in the moment:

- **Observe:** Pay attention to events/experiences, thoughts, emotions, and behavior without trying to change anything.
- **Describe:** Use your words to describe the event/experience and your response.
- **Participate:** Engage in the moment without feeling self-conscious.

How skills

How skills refer to how you observe, describe, and participate:

- **Non-judgmental:** Avoid attaching a label to an event/experience (e.g., it is "good" or "bad").
- **Mindful:** Be present in the moment. This means you are not multitasking!
- **Effective:** Do what you need to do using practical or efficient means

Handout 4.3: A Balanced Approach

Using a balanced approach in life encourages us to look at problem areas in our lives and create balance. "Balance" refers to the ability to maintain a life that feels stable. In other words, it allows you to navigate your life without falling, or to quickly "bounce back" after falling. But balance in our lives requires us to practice balancing our thoughts, feelings, and associated behaviors.

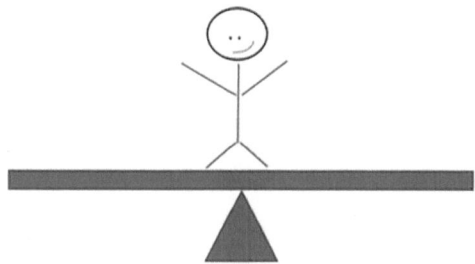

Desire to escape the moment/ feeling	**Radical acceptance of the moment**
Allow yourself to be aware of your discomfort in the moment AND accept the moment for what it is.	

Reduce negative emotions	**Trust own emotions**
Allow yourself to recognize negative emotions when they arise AND acknowledge that that feelings are not facts.	

Feelings of powerlessness Feeling powerful

Allow yourself to be vulnerable AND recognize the parts of your life you have power.

Desire for intimacy   Desire for autonomy

Allow yourself to have intimacy in your life AND make time for yourself.

Other?

Handout 4.4: FLOURISH Skills for Living a Wise Life

Remembering the acronym FLOURISH can help remind you to build more positive connections in your brain. The acronym stands for:

- **F**ind silver linings.
- **L**ive mindfully.
- **O**ffer self-compassion.
- **U**se positive self-talk.
- **R**elate (i.e., build social connections).
- **I**gnite passions.
- **S**hift your focus to the positive.
- **H**old gratitude in order to create a life worth living.

F: <u>Find silver linings</u> means trying to find helpful lessons in negative situations. This helps us focus on the positive side of things.

Example: Prison has been very difficult for Jesús. He is three years into a 10-year sentence. As awful as it is to be away from his family, living in a dangerous, confined environment, Jesús can continue drawing, writing, and sending his art to his loved ones on the outside.

L: <u>Living mindfully</u> means paying attention to what is happening right now, without judging it. It helps us learn to enjoy the good moments more, notice good feelings in our bodies, and be present in the moment.

Example: Jesús practices living mindfully when he is completely engaged in his artwork and writing. He notices feelings of calm, excitement, and contentment when he is working on his art.

O: <u>Offering self-compassion</u> means being kind to ourselves. It means treating ourselves with care and understanding, especially when things are hard.

Example: Pierre was just denied parole for the second time. Despite feeling disappointed, he reminds himself that he committed a violent crime, and that the parole board does not typically grant men who have committed sexual offenses parole at their first or second hearings. Pierre acknowledges his feelings about his current situation, accepts them, and gives himself permission to take a short nap.

U: <u>Using positive self-talk</u> refers to the positive things we tell ourselves about ourselves.

Example: Pierre tells himself that he will be eligible for parole in another three years, and that there are things he can do during that time to make himself a better candidate for early release.

R: Relating, or building positive social connections, means making an effort to have good relationships with others. When we spend time with people whom we care about, and when we support each other, it makes us feel that we are not alone.

Example: Andre has just been released from prison and does not have a supportive family or friend circle. He feels alone in the world and wishes he had positive connections with others. His therapist asks him about his interests and helps him find low-cost/free groups in the community with other likeminded individuals whom he can interact with.

I: Igniting passions means finding and engaging in activities that bring us joy. This helps enhance overall happiness and satisfaction.

Example: Andre actively attends group meetups at a comedy club and begins learning how to write his own comedy material.

S: Shifting the focus away from negative thoughts to thoughts that are more helpful and effective. When we use thought stopping, or thought shifting, we can disrupt negative self-talk.

Example: The last two women that Jonah took on a date "ghosted" him afterwards. Jonah feels rejected and lonely, but reminds himself that dating is difficult, and it typically takes many tries before meeting a person with whom one is compatible. He remembers his therapist's words that "there's someone out there for everyone."

H: Holding gratitude refers to the practice of intentionally acknowledging and appreciating the present moment with a sense of openness and non-judgment. It involves developing an attitude of genuine appreciation for the positive aspects of our lives, no matter how big or small they may be.

Example: Perry does not have a car, so he has to walk 20 minutes home with his groceries for the week. The groceries are heavy, and it is hot and humid outside; but Perry is grateful that he is no longer incarcerated, and that he can choose his own food, and walk freely in his community.

Notes

1 Sakdalan & Gupta (2014).
2 R. Hanson (2013).
3 Kabat-Zinn (2018).
4 Skaldalan & Gupta (2012).

References

Hanson R. (2013). *Hardwiring Happiness: The New Brain Science of Contentment, Calm, and Confidence.* Unabridged. New York: Random House Audio.

Kabat-Zinn J. (2018). *Falling Awake: How to Practice Mindfulness in Everyday Life.* New York: Hatchett Books.

Sakdalan J. A. & Gupta R. (2012). Wise mind–risky mind: A reconceptualisation of dialectical behaviour therapy concepts and its application to sexual offender treatment.*JournalofSexualAggression,20*(1),110–120.https://.doi.10.1080/13552600. 2012.723357

Part II
Sexual Regulation Skills

Healthy Sexuality, Intrusive Thoughts, and Compulsive Behaviors

5

The second part of dialectical behavioral therapy (DBT) skills training addresses sexual dysregulation—specifically the role of deviant fantasies, the use of sex to cope with emotions, and the factors that led to the offense. Teaching healthy sexuality is important for many reasons. First, clients are familiarized with healthy and unhealthy sexual practices of which they may not have been aware. This is particularly important for clients who did not receive much, if any, sexual education. Second, these discussions facilitate a more open atmosphere, which leads to a higher comfort level discussing sex and sexuality. Third, clients gain a deeper awareness of their own perceptions of sexuality and how these perceptions led to their offending behavior.

At this point, group members will be asked to disclose their offense to the group so that they have a more meaningful understanding of one another, and can respectfully challenge one another's thinking errors for the duration of treatment. This step also often helps to alleviate shame and increase group cohesion.

Disclosure can be a challenging and emotional experience for clients, as they will be asked to share their offense(s) with a group of people. It is common for clients to leave out important information about their offense (minimizing). While this is expected, it is important to avoid colluding with the client. As such, if the client has finished sharing their disclosure statement but has not addressed the specific aspects of their offense, gently prompt them. It helps to first let them know they are off to a "good start," but that there is more information that is important for the group to know about

DOI: 10.4324/9781003451099-8

the offense in order to support the client throughout treatment. You may consider asking follow-up questions such as, "What happened before/after ...?," "What were the factors that motivated you to begin offending in the first place?," or "What motivated you to continue offending even though you knew it was illegal?"

> **Skills Trainer:**
> *Some people are attracted to minors or other illegal sexual behaviors. If you have always had, for example, an attraction to minors, you may have had difficulty becoming aroused by an adult partner. This has posed problems for you in the past, which is why you are here. A predisposition of attraction to minors is frustrating for many men because it is illegal to have sex with those to whom they are attracted. Many men who have such an attraction also feel shame, and hence are reluctant to disclose the attraction to anyone.*
>
> *It is fairly common that people who have committed a sexual offense lack a firm understanding of sex, sexuality, or their bodies. The purpose of talking about sexual regulation skills is to help you become more familiar with normative sexual thoughts and behavior, and be able to recognize when you are having sexual thoughts that put you at risk of reoffending.*

Explain that one's understanding of sex and sexuality are initially shaped by factors such as culture, family, and community; however, it is also shaped through interactions with others, and thoughts based on individual experiences.[1] Thus, it is important to teach clients about the various components of healthy sexuality, and the skills needed to regulate problematic sexual behaviors, while maintaining an open, culturally competent view of clients' understanding.

Prior to teaching sexual regulation skills, it is useful to find out what clients know and do not know about healthy sexuality. Ask participants to take out Handout 5.1: What Is Healthy Sexuality? and ask them to list words or phrases they associate with healthy sexuality, and those they associate with unhealthy sexuality. Once they have completed this, group members should share the words on their list and the skills trainer should write them on a whiteboard or large piece of paper. You will likely notice that some clients' beliefs about healthy sexuality are inaccurate, misguided, or potentially illegal (e.g., "rough," "men dominate," "as long as they're 16, it's legal," etc.).

After the lists have been completed, ask clients what differences they notice between the two lists. After discussing the lists, you can talk to clients about general, normative definitions of unhealthy and healthy sexuality. These points might make sense to your clients in theory, but many will be left wondering how they can employ skills to attain healthy sexual wellbeing.

Skills Trainer: Give clients approximately 10 minutes to make a list of their understanding of "healthy sexuality," and "unhealthy sexuality" (Handout 5.1: What Is Healthy Sexuality?). Once they have completed their lists, encourage group discussion about their perceptions.

Discuss the worksheets with the group. Explain that sexual health does not just include absence of disease; it also plays an important role in one's physical, emotional, and social wellbeing, and thus a more balanced life. In fact, someone may not achieve an erection and/or ejaculate all the time. This is normal; however, if it is happening often, or "out of the blue," it is important to take a step back and consider physical and psychological reasons this might be happening. Of note, clients often ask me questions about difficulty getting or maintaining an erection. I typically respond by explaining that the reasons could be biological, emotional/psychological, or behavioral. Aging, injury, and medication can all play a role in a man's ability to get or stay erect or achieve an orgasm. It is important to see a medical doctor if the client notices sudden changes in their sexual arousal patterns.

Often, men who experience this issue feel inadequate, ashamed, and/ or unworthy. However, inability to achieve or maintain an erection, or ejaculate need not impede an individual from engaging in healthy sexual activity with his partner(s). Suggestions you can offer your clients for sexual intimacy without having an erection include kissing, touching, oral sex, anal play, or consensual kinky play (e.g., handcuffs, blindfolds, feathers, or ice cubes).

Can you think of other ways to be sexually intimate without having an erection?

Consider the nature of your relationship with your sexual partner. Are you physically and sexually attracted to them? Physical attraction plays a large role in sexual arousal. In fact, a number of men say that they are worried that they cannot achieve an erection with their sexual partner. When questioned further about the nature of their relationship, they may admit that they are no longer physically attracted to their partner because their partner has gained a significant amount of weight, or experienced other physical changes that they find unappealing.

Encourage clients to use effective means to address this problem.

Telling your partner that you are not physically attracted to them because their appearance has changed is not helpful and may lead to conflict between the two of you. Imagine if your partner told you that they do not find you attractive anymore. How would you feel? There are other ways you can address this issue in a respectful way. Instead, you can ask your partner to take walks or bike rides together, or engage in other physical activities with you. You can say, "I would really like to spend more quality time with you and get out of the house. Let's go for a walk together." Ask your partner to have a "date" with you that involves dressing somewhat less casually than on a normal day. The date does not need to be "fancy," or involve spending lots of money. For example, you could prepare a picnic for you and your partner. You could also try creating a consensual sexual roleplay experience at home, or a movie night at home.

Changes in physical appearance, however, are not the only source of decreased sexual attraction to one's partner. Many clients share that their relationship is chaotic, unstable, and/or includes frequent arguments.

Skills Trainer:
Chaotic relationships can take a toll on someone's desire to be intimate with their partner because they do not feel emotionally connected or emotionally safe. This issue is a bit more difficult to address because something deeper than physical attraction is going on in your relationship. We will discuss this more when we learn about intimacy; however, let's brainstorm ideas that you can use if you find yourself in this situation.

If clients are having a difficult a time brainstorming, you can recommend the following:

- Scheduling time to have a "sit-down" discussion with your partner about your feelings and concerns. Remember that this is not just about your personal feelings and concerns, but also about theirs. Ask them how they feel about the relationship, what they enjoy about the relationship, and what they would like to change. Are these changes feasible/manageable? If so, commit to working on these changes with your partner.
- Schedule couples counseling if possible. This could include counseling from a mental health professional, a religious/spiritual leader in your community, or a community-based workshop.
- If changes are not feasible, it is worth considering whether the relationship can withstand this issue.
- Finally, if the relationship is toxic and not contributing to your wise life, you may want to consider ending it.

Skills Trainer:
Some men have trouble achieving an erection with a partner because they spend too much time viewing pornography and masturbating to it.

Ask clients to brainstorm ideas to address this issue. Be sure to encourage them to make a list of various interests or hobbies they can pursue when the urge to watch pornography, and/or masturbate arises.

> *While some masturbation is normal, doing it too frequently can lead to difficulty becoming erect or having an orgasm with your partner.*

Skills Trainer:
Another reason why some men have trouble achieving an erection with a partner is because they fear sexual intimacy. This is specifically relevant for individuals that are used to having frequent "hook-ups," or that avoid sexual intimacy altogether. Talking to your therapist is the most important way to address this issue. They can assist you in gaining insight into your fear and avoidance. If you tend to have frequent casual sex with others, it might be a good idea to stop placing yourself in situations where you have access to multiple and/or unknown potential sexual partners. Instead, create a list of things you can do when you feel the urge to have sex with someone, or when you feel lonely.

Group Discussion: Ask clients why they believe sex is part of a wise life. Next, draw a line down the center of the whiteboard to create two columns: "pros" and "cons." Ask clients to list the pros and cons of building a life with a sexual partner versus having casual sex.

Intrusive Thoughts and Compulsive Behavior

It is important to distinguish between sexual thoughts and sexual fantasies involving illegal scenarios.[2] Intrusive thoughts are not necessarily the result of a deliberate desire to fantasize about legal or illegal sexual behavior; nor do they necessarily lead to acting out. However, an individual does have the ability to disrupt or "thought stop" before the thought begins to spiral out of control. One of the main goals of DBT is to teach clients how to stop automatic thoughts before they lead to fantasies involving illegal scenarios. These types of sexual fantasies are the result of intentionally generated scenarios, [3] which may include memories of one's own victimization, memories of victimizing others, [4] or thoughts about future offending.[5] Moreover, these types of sexual fantasies have the potential to place individuals at risk of future reoffending because they elicit sexual arousal that may lead to masturbation, thus conditioning these scenarios and leading the individual to desire acting them out.

Scholars have shown that people learn to masturbate to deviant sexual fantasies by experiencing and then reenacting the behavior, viewing various types of media and engaging in previous deviant contact, masturbation to deviant fantasies, or visual representations of deviant behavior—all of which has the potential to reinforce the unhealthy thoughts and possibly perpetuate reoffending.[6] The main point is that unhealthy sexual fantasies may become a focus when an individual experiences negative emotions such as rejection, powerlessness, shame, despair, hopelessness, helplessness, or fear.[7]

We often hear clients report that their offending was the result of a sex or pornography "addiction." This may be true in part; however, it is important to define the term "addiction," and ensure your clients do not use this as an excuse for offending. While "sexual addiction" is not listed as an addiction in the *Diagnostic and Statistical Manual of Mental Disorders, Fifth Edition*, Kafka (2010)[8] has identified factors that define "sexual addiction" as follows:

- The individual spends more time engaging in sexual fantasy and behavior than addressing their daily responsibilities.
- The compulsive behavior is initiated when the individual experiences negative emotions or a difficult event.
- The individual is unable to stop despite attempts to do so.
- The individual's behavior poses a threat or risk to themselves or others.

While sexual addiction is not always implicated in sexual offending,[9] there are some similarities between sexual compulsivity among sexual offenders and non-offenders,[10] such as ritualistic and cyclical behavior.[11] This means that sexual offenders often begin their chain of offending by masturbating to deviant sexual fantasies, or engaging in routines in anticipation of offending (e.g., grooming, use/increased use of drugs or alcohol, and spending time in certain areas such as parks or playgrounds).[12] As such, I replace the term "sexual addiction" with "sexual compulsivity."

Research has shown that both classical and operant conditioning are implicated in the acquisition of deviant sexual arousal patterns. As such, the best way to decrease these arousal patterns is to use reconditioning techniques.[13] Aversive techniques such as odor aversion, directed masturbation, and development of appropriate sexual fantasy can all be useful behavioral interventions; however, caution is warranted, as research has demonstrated mixed results regarding the use of these techniques.[14]

Skills Trainer: Begin by asking the group to define what "intrusive thoughts" are and to provide examples. Next, ask them to define and provide examples of "compulsive behaviors."

Intrusive thoughts are recurring unwanted or unhelpful thoughts, impulses, or images that pop into our heads. While they may pop up randomly, they often have been conditioned, or triggered, by something one saw, heard, tasted, smelled, experienced, or thought in the past. Once these thoughts arise, they can be difficult to get rid of; and oftentimes people find themselves going down the proverbial rabbit hole.

Group Discussion: Ask clients to share a time when they had an intrusive thought that led to more intrusive thoughts and eventually to illegal behavior. If their examples do not include their offense, ask them to consider what kinds of intrusive thoughts they had prior to and during their offending. Explain that it is normal for people to have sexual fantasies about engaging in legal sexual behavior. However, the problem arises when an individual is using their sexual fantasies as an escape from dealing with their problems, or is fantasizing about engaging in illegal sexual behavior.

Next, explain that the clients will complete Handout 5.2: My Intrusive Thoughts and Compulsive Behaviors. For this assignment, they should list common intrusive thoughts and compulsive behaviors, both sexual and non-sexual. Do not ask them to elaborate on the thoughts or behaviors, as this could potentially arouse them. If the client tends to become preoccupied by their problematic thoughts and behaviors, you may ask them to complete the homework with their individual counselor, and/or make sure they have ammonia or another aversive smell handy (e.g., deer urine, rotten meat in a container) while they complete the assignment.

Handout 5.1: What is Healthy Sexuality?

List the words that you associate with *healthy* sexuality:

1. _____
2. _____
3. _____
4. _____
5. _____
6. _____
7. _____
8. _____
9. _____
10. _____

Now, list the words you associate with *unhealthy* sexuality:

1. _____
2. _____
3. _____
4. _____
5. _____
6. _____
7. _____
8. _____
9. _____
10. _____

Handout 5.2: My Intrusive Thoughts and Compulsive Behaviors

Everyone has experienced intrusive thoughts at some point in their lives. These thoughts are recurring and cause distress. For this assignment, make a list of intrusive thoughts you have experienced or currently experience. These thoughts should include sexual thoughts, although it is helpful also to list other, non-sexual thoughts that have created problems for you in the past or currently.

In the second box, list the behaviors that you engaged in after each intrusive thought. For example, your intrusive thought might be about engaging in sex with a minor. The behavior that followed the thought might include you viewing child pornography, or going to a park to look at children.

If you need more space, write on the back of this page.

Intrusive thought	Accompanying behavior

Notes

1 Gagnon (1990).
2 I avoid the term "deviant," as it is associated with deficits-based treatment models that emphasize a confrontational approach. Research has consistently demonstrated that approaching treatment from a deficit perspective is ineffective in creating motivation for change, and ultimately reducing recidivism (e.g., see Marshall, 2019).
3 Byers, Purdon, & Clark (1998).
4 Gee, Ward, Belofastov, & Beeck (2006).
5 Beech & Bartels (2016); Delmonico, Griffin, & Carnes (2002).
6 Laws & Marshall (1990).
7 Delmonico, Griffin, & Carnes (2002).
8 Kafka (2010) argues that three of these factors must be present over a period of six months or more to qualify as a sexual addiction.
9 Giordano (2022). In fact, in Marshall et al.'s (2008) study of incarcerated sexual offenders found that 43.9% of sexual offenders met their criteria for a sexual addiction.
10 Delmonico, Griffin, & Carnes (2002).
11 Giordano (2022); Delmonico, Griffin, & Carnes (2002).
12 See Wolf's (1988) cycle of offending.
13 Aytes, Olsen, Zakrajsek, Murray, & Ireson (2001).
14 See, Burke, Dwyer, & Riesling (2014); Campbell-Fuller & Craig (2009); McGrath (1991).

References

Aytes K. E., Olsen S. S., Zakrajsek T., Murray P., & Ireson R. (2001). Cognitive/behavioral treatment for sexual offenders: An examination of recidivism. *Sexual Abuse*, 13(4), 223–231. https://doi.org/10.1023/A:1017552514037

Beech A., & Bartels R. (2016). Theories of deviant sexual fantasy. In Boer D. P. (ed.), *The Wiley Blackwell Handbook on Assessment, Treatment and Theories of Sexual Offending*, Volume 1. New York: Wiley.

Burke W., Dwyer G., & Riesling C. (2014) Using behavioral techniques to control sexual arousal. In Carich M. S., & Mussack, S. E. (eds.), *The Safer Society Handbook of Sexual Abuser Assessment and Treatment*. Brandon, VT: The Safer Society Press.

Byers E. S., Purdon, C., & Clark, D. A. (1998) Sexual intrusive thoughts of college students, The *Journal of Sex Research*, 35(4), 359–369. https://doi.org/10.1080/00224499809551954

Campbell-Fuller N., & Craig L.A. (2009). The use of olfactory aversion and directed masturbation in modifying deviant sexual interest: a case study. *Journal of Sexual Aggression*, 15(2), 171–191.

Delmonico D. L., Griffin E., & Carnes P. J. (2002). Treating online compulsive sexual behavior: When cybersex is the drug of choice. In Cooper A. (ed.), *Sex and the Internet: A Guidebook for Clinicians* (pp. 147–167). New York: Brunner-Routledge.

Gee D., Ward T., Belofastov A., & Beech A. (2006). The structural properties of sexual fantasies for sexual offenders: A preliminary model. *Journal of Sexual Aggression, 12*(3), 2013–226. https://doi.org/10.1080/13552600601009956

Giordano A. L. (2022). *A Clinical Guide to Treating Behavioral Addictions: Conceptualizations, Assessments, and Clinical Strategies.* New York: Springer Publishing Company.

Kafka M. P. (2010). Hypersexual disorder: A proposed diagnosis for DSM-V. *Archives of Sexual Behavior, 39,* 377–400. https://doi.org/10.1007/s10508-009-9574-7

Laws D. R., & Marshall W. L. (1990). A conditioning theory of the etiology and maintenance of deviant sexual preference and behavior. In Marshall W. L., Laws D. R., & Barbaree H. E. (eds.), *Handbook of Sexual Assault: Issues, Theories, and Treatment of the Offender* (pp. 209–229). Boston, MA: Plenum Press.

Marshall, L.E. (2019). Effective sex offender treatment in correctional settings: A strengths-based approach. In Polaschek D.L., A, & Hollin C.R. (eds.), *The Wiley International Handbook of Correctional Psychology.* Hoboken, NJ: John Wiley & Sons Ltd.

Gagnon J. H. (1990). The explicit and implicit use of the scripting perspective in sex research. *Annual Review of Sex Research, 1,* 1–43. https://doi.org/10.1080/105325 28.1990.10559854

Marshall L. E., Marshall W. L., Moulden H. M., & Serran G. A. (2008). The prevalence of 33 sexual addiction in incarcerated sexual offenders and matched community nonoffenders. *Sexual Addiction and Compulsivity, 15*(4), 271–283. https://doi.org/10.1080/10720160802516328

McGrath R. J. (1991). Sex-offender risk assessment and disposition planning: A review of empirical and clinical findings. *International Journal of Offender Therapy and Comparative Criminology, 35*(4), 328–350. https://doi.org/10.1177/0306624X9103500407

Wolf S.C. (1988) A model of sexual aggression/addiction. *Journal of Social Work and Human Sexuality, 7*(1), 131–148. https://doi.org/10.1300/J291v07n01_10

CALM and CLASP Skills   **6**

Skills Trainer:

We have discussed how sexual fantasies about engaging in illegal behavior play a role in sexual offending. However, there are more components that lead to this behavior that, if addressed, can help men charged with these offences from reoffending. Review, in detail, the CALM and CLASP skills (Handouts 6.1: CALM Skills and 6.3: CLASP Skills).

- _**C**onversation:_ *Before engaging in sexual play with someone, make sure you are in agreement about your sexual likes and dislikes. If the other person is uncomfortable with particular sexual behaviors, you must respect that. Do not try to "convince" the other person to do something they do not want to do."*

Group Discussion: Having conversations about sex, and sexual interests and dislikes, is awkward for many people. Elicit some ideas from group members that they can use when having these conversations.

- _**A**void Pornography:_ *Many men who commit sexual offences have viewed a significant amount of pornography, legal and illegal. Even if you currently or used to view legal pornography, you probably know that it is a "slippery slope" and leads to regular viewing, especially when you masturbate and orgasm to the images. Pornography also contains elements of misogyny (demonstrating contempt for, or prejudice against women; objectification of women). In addition, because it is unrealistic, viewers*

DOI: 10.4324/9781003451099-9

often have the wrong idea about what sex "should" look like, what the other person wants to do, and what others enjoy sexually.

- **Learn your arousal patterns:** *What arouses you, specifically? It is important to be aware of one's sexual interests, and to manage them appropriately and legally. Some people become aroused by legal situations, while others are aroused by illegal situations. When individuals are aroused by children/minors, animals, inflicting harm on a non-consenting person, exposing themselves in public, rubbing up against non-consenting people, or any other illegal sexual behavior, it is important to recognize it in order to avoid reoffending.*

Group Discussion: Give clients five minutes to write a list of what arouses them. Make sure they also discuss this list with their individual therapist.

- **Masturbation:** *It is important to consider how masturbation plays a role in healthy and problematic sexuality. People convicted of sexual offences have typically masturbated to fantasies about illegal behavior. These fantasies have been conditioned or learned. In other words, an individual's desire to watch pornography is reinforced by his orgasm.*

Note: For example, child sexual exploitation material (CSEM) offenders typically begin viewing adult pornography, fantasize about these images, and masturbate to them. Frequent viewing of and fantasizing about legal pornography eventually become monotonous for these offenders. As arousal to these images decreases, they begin to search for more risqué or deviant materials, such as pornography depicting bestiality; bondage, discipline, sadism and masochism; sexual activity involving excrement; and eventually videos and images of child sexual exploitation. As the individual's viewing of CSEM escalates, offenders will often fantasize about child sexual exploitation and masturbate to these fantasies, thus reinforcing their arousal to them.

Group Discussion: Ask clients to look at Handout 6.2: What Is Appropriate Masturbation? For this activity, clients will have 10 minutes to create a list of sexual fantasies that are not appropriate; that they are unsure whether or not are appropriate; and that are appropriate. Once they have completed their lists, ask each participant to share their list. Create three columns on the whiteboard and record participants' responses. You may notice that some participants confuse healthy with unhealthy. Be sure to have a discussion about normative and non-normative masturbatory patterns after clients have completed the activity.

Skills Trainer: Explain that everyone has a worldview that has been constructed by their interactions with other people, situations, and experiences. This is referred to as a "schema," but "framework" might be an easier term for clients to understand and visualize.

We will continue to learn more skills for healthy sexual practices that specifically rely on your social interactions with potential sexual partners. These are the CLASP skills.

The various factors that construct our worldview are important because they help us understand why we think, feel, and behave the way we do. Conversely, not understanding these factors can lead to problems identifying situations that cause us to behave ineffectively, illegally, or in a harmful way. Understanding your sexual schema is an important component of sex offender treatment because it encourages you to think about your own sexuality, sexual attitudes, beliefs, feelings, and behaviors, and how they have influenced your life and relationships.

Ask clients to consider their own sexual framework during this week as they complete their homework, Handout 6.5: My Sexual Framework.

Handout 6.1: CALM Skills

- **Conversation:** Before engaging in sexual play with someone, make sure you are in agreement about your sexual likes and dislikes. If the other person is uncomfortable with particular sexual behaviors, you must respect that. Do not try to "convince" the other person to do something they do not want to do.
- **Avoid pornography:** Even legal pornography can be a "slippery slope" and lead to regular viewing.
- **Learn your arousal patterns:** It is important to be aware of one's sexual interests, and to manage them appropriately and legally.
- **Masturbation:** It is important to consider how masturbation plays a role in your sexuality. What types of situations or fantasies sexually arouse you? If these include illegal situations, or deviant sexual fantasies, refer to Handout 6.2: Appropriate Masturbation.

Homework: What is Appropriate Masturbation?

Image 6.1 Red Octogon

1. _____
2. _____
3. _____
4. _____

5. _____
6. _____
7. _____
8. _____
9. _____
10. _____

???

1. _____
2. _____
3. _____
4. _____
5. _____
6. _____
7. _____
8. _____
9. _____
10. _____

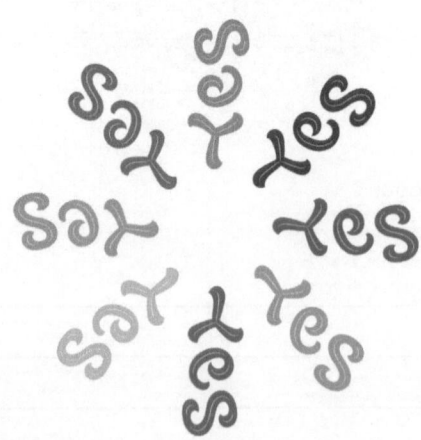

Image 6.2 Yes circles

1. _____

2. _____

3. _____

4. _____

5. _____

6. _____

7. _____

8. _____

9. _____

10. _____

Handout 6.2: Appropriate Masturbation

You should never masturbate to illegal fantasies. If you are having an illegal fantasy, do not allow yourself to ejaculate to it. The following is a list of things you can practice to ensure healthy masturbation.

- STOP! Do not continue to masturbate to an unhealthy/illegal fantasy.
- Do something different. You can do the following to reduce your arousal:
    - Use odor aversion (e.g., ammonia, rotten meat, or deer urine).
    - Take a cold shower.
    - Put ice on your wrists.
    - Put ice in a towel and place it on your genitals for 20 seconds.
    - Call someone.
    - Pinch yourself/place a rubber band around your wrist and snap it.
    - Go for a walk.
    - Complete a behavior chain analysis.
- Tell yourself "Switch" or "Change the channel" and change your thoughts to your appropriate fantasy.
- Tell yourself "Switch" or "Change the channel" and proceed with mindful masturbation.
- Other ideas?.

_____

_____

_____

_____

_____

Handout 6.3: CLASP Skills

- **Consent/ Legal:** Oftentimes, people are not completely aware of the rules surrounding consent for sexual activity. It is important to remember that you must obtain consent with any sexual partner, including your spouse. The following is a list of rules of consent:
    - Consent and legal sexual activity include asking the other person if they want to have sex with you.
    - "No" means no.
    - Silence/absence of "yes" means no.
    - Remember that consent is required for each sexual activity. Your partner may want to stop at a certain point. You must stop, even if you have already penetrated your partner.
    - If your partner has asked you to wear a condom, you must wear a condom before penetrating them. You cannot remove the condom during sexual activity without their permission.
    - A person who is under the influence of drugs or alcohol cannot consent.
    - A sleeping person cannot consent.
    - Someone who is passed out cannot consent.
    - A person with an intellectual disability cannot consent.
    - A person who is clearly displaying psychiatric problems cannot consent.
    - An animal cannot consent.
    - In Georgia, the age of consent for sexual activity is 16 years. In other states, it is 18 years. It is your responsibility to be aware of this. Believing someone is 16 years or older (i.e., "But she looked like an adult") is not an excuse in the eyes of the law. You will be held accountable for your actions.

Note: Be mindful of differences in power (e.g., having sex with your employee, student, etc.). This could be very problematic for you.

- **Ask age:** Verify your date or sexual partner's age by asking for identification.
- **Step-by-step interactions:** Pay attention to your interaction with the other person. Individuals—especially women—often do not want to appear rude, so they may not outright tell you they do not want to talk

to you. If someone does not want to talk to or engage with you, it is important to accept that without berating the other person, or calling them names. Remember: you are not interested in everyone who is interested in you, and not everyone you are interested in is available or interested in you.

- The following behaviors are typically uncomfortable for others:
  - Standing too close to the other person/invading their physical boundary.
  - Oversharing personal information.
  - Asking personal information when you do not know the person well.
  - Making sexual references to someone with whom you are not in a relationship; talking about sex.
  - Touching the other person's body without consent. Be mindful that many people—especially women—have experienced some type of sexual violation and do not feel comfortable when strangers touch them. Depending on the situation, this may constitute sexual battery.
  - Not leaving someone alone when they ask you to.
  - Yelling, swearing, or threatening someone who has indicated they want to be left alone.
- The following behaviors in someone else probably indicate that they are not interested in having a conversation with you:
  - They give short responses, do not ask you questions, do not appear engaged in the conversation, or feign laughter.
  - They refuse to make eye contact, turn away from you, talk to others instead of you, or look at their phone.
  - They back up/away from you.
- **Protection:** Be sure to use protection when you engage in oral, anal, or vaginal intercourse with another person. If you have a long-term partner, getting tested for sexually transmitted infections is also wise.

Handout 6.4: Unhealthy and Illegal Sexual Behaviors

- Lack of communication.
- Lack of consent.
- Lying to your partner(s).
- Disrespecting your partner(s).
- Hurting others.
- Exploiting others.
- Compulsive sexuality.
- Not practicing safe sex.
- Viewing sex as shameful/dirty.
- Emotional distance from partner(s).
- Sex with strangers.

Skills for healthy sexual wellbeing[1]

- Ability to communicate open and honestly about sex, sexuality, needs, and desires when you and the other person are ready. Examples include:
  - "How do you feel about me?" "Are you interested in me physically?" "Are you attracted to me? "Would you like to kiss?" "What are your sexual preferences?" "May I kiss you?" "What do you not enjoy?" "What do you need from me to feel comfortable?" "I do/do not enjoy…." "I like it when …"
  - "I have/have not been tested recently—how about you?"
  - Discussion of medical issues such as erectile dysfunction or sexually transmitted infections.
- Ability to initiate consensual sex. Examples include:
  - "Do you want to have sex?" "Let me know what you would like me to do."
  - Asking your sexual partner(s) if they are comfortable at each stage (e.g., taking off clothing, touching genitals, penetration, etc.).
- Ability to say "no" when you do not want sex. Examples include:
  - "I'm not really feeling it today. Rain check?"
  - "I'd like to get to know you a little better first."

- Ability to accept when someone does not want to have sex. Examples include:
  - "I understand." "No problem." "Let me know if or when you feel comfortable."
  - Asking if they would like to do something else (sexual or non-sexual).
  - Avoiding being passive-aggressive (e.g., "Well, fine then"), "pushy," angry, violent, or telling them that they are being a "tease."
- Acceptance of the other person's decision that they do not want to have sex with you. In other words, you accept that "no means no," and do not attempt to pressure or guilt the other person into changing their mind.
  - Ability to respect boundaries – your own and those of others. Examples include:
  - "I'm not comfortable doing that." "I'd like to get to know you a little better first."
- Getting to know your sexual partner(s).
- Consent, equality, respect, trust, safety (CERTS).

Handout 6.5: My Sexual Framework

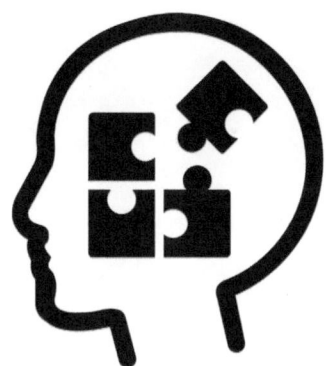

Image 6.3 Head with puzzle pieces for brain

Cultural: Cultural norms, values, expectations, and rules about sex/sexuality. The individual learns what they can/cannot do (e.g., in religious households there are often stigmas around pre-marital sex, masturbation, and other forms of sexual expression.

Internal: A person's understanding of physical, emotional, and cognitive cues associated with sex (e.g., "If I am feeling aroused then I have to do something about it" such as view pornography, masturbate, have sex).

Interpersonal: Cues perceived by an individual that lead them to believe another person is interested in sex. Those beliefs then drive the individual's behavior (e.g., "She's wearing a short skirt and low-cut shirt, so she's looking to have sex).

- List the healthy sexual behaviors you practice/have engaged in.
- List the unhealthy sexual behaviors you practice/ have engaged in.
- How have the following factors influenced your beliefs about sex and sexuality?
  - Culture.
  - Community.
  - Family.
  - Religion/spirituality.

- Friends.
- Intimate relationships.
- Traumatic experiences.
- What would you like to do differently to promote your healthy sexual wellbeing?

Note

1   Maltz & Holman (1987); Marshall et al. (2016); Watter & Hall (2020).

References

Maltz W., & Holman B. (1987). *Incest and Sexuality: A Guide to Understanding and Healing.* Washington, D.C.: Lexington Books.

Marshall W. L., Hall K. S., & Woo C P. (2016). Sexual functioning in the treatment of sex offenders. In Boer D. P. (ed.). *The Wiley Handbook on the Theories, Assessment and Treatment of Sexual Offending:* New York: Wiley.

Watter D. N., Hall K. S. K. (2020). Healthy sexuality for sex offenders. *Current Psychiatry Reports 22*(55). https://doi.org/10.1007/s11920-020-01180-1

Thinking Errors and Risk Factors 7

It is important to acknowledge that most people do not simply decide to commit a sexual offense one day. While people's metacognitions may not have kicked in during their offending period, they were nonetheless aware of the illegal nature of their behavior. As with people who commit other offenses, those who commit sexual offenses have a tendency to resort to cognitive distortions (thinking errors) to rationalize, minimize, or justify their behavior. It is important that clients can identify the type of thinking error(s) they typically have, and especially the thinking errors leading up to the offense, and post-offense.

> **Skills Trainer:**
> *Take a look at Handout 7.1: Thinking Errors, which lists common thinking errors that many people have at some point in their lives. Thinking errors are defined as "a thought that is not true," or "an unhelpful thought." Some people have more different types of thinking errors than others, and some people have thinking errors more often than others. In general, people use thinking errors to:*
> - *Justify their actions.*
> - *Minimize their actions.*
> - *Rationalize their actions.*
>
> *This is particularly true of individuals who have committed sexual offenses. It is important to identify the type of thinking error(s) you are prone to, and when you are having one.*

DOI: 10.4324/9781003451099-10

Review Handout 7.1: Thinking Errors in detail with the group.

Skills Trainer: Keep in mind that there are specific thinking errors ("implicit theories") identified by the literature that increase the likelihood of offending for different types of offenders. If group members fail to identify these, be sure to add them to the list.

> *Common thinking errors among men who sexually abuse children include the following:* [1]
> - **Children are sexual beings:** *This refers to the idea that children want to learn about sex/sexuality from you; they are being flirtatious with you; pubescent teens in pornography are "enjoying" what they are doing because they are smiling.*
> - **Nature of harm:** *Sexual contact between kids and adults is harmless unless there is violence.*
>   - *"I wasn't hurting her; I was teaching her how to kiss/have sex."*
>   - *"I was teaching him what love feels like."*
> - **Uncontrollability:** *The belief that your basic needs are driving the offense and you cannot control your urges.*
>   - *"Men are sexual beings. We want sex all the time."*
>   - *"It's in our genes."*
>   - *"I have a porn/sex addiction."*
>   - *"It's human nature. The Greeks and Romans did it thousands of years ago and it wasn't illegal then. Our society is too uptight about sex."*
> - **Entitlement:** *The belief that you can behave the way you want because you are superior.*
>   - *"I deserve to touch her because I had a hard day at work."*
>   - *"I don't care about my restrictions. I should have the right to sit near the playground."*
>   - *"I am an adult. Children should respect adults ... no matter what."*
> - **Dangerous world:** *The belief that danger exists all around you and the best way to deal with a hostile world is to take control/dominate situations.*
>   - *"That little boy's mom isn't watching him. She doesn't care what happens to him. I will go over there and talk to him to teach her a lesson."*
>   - *"Adults are so judgmental, but kids really 'get' me. They don't judge."*
> *Common thinking errors among men who have committed rape include the following:* [2]
> - **Women are unknowable:** *The belief that women are fundamentally different from men, or try to deceive men.*

- o   *"Men are from Mars; women are from Venus."*
- o   *"Women play mind games with men."*
- **Women are sex objects:** *All women want sex from men, even if they don't know they do.*
  - o   *"Men can tell when a woman 'wants it' by her body language, clothing, or language."*
- **The male sex drive is uncontrollable:** *When men become aroused, they simply can't control themselves.*
  - o   *"Men think with their genitals, not their brains."*
- **Entitlement:** *The belief that men's needs should be met on demand.*
  - o   *"I can take what I want, when I want it."*
  - o   *"Everyone does what's in their best interests anyway, so why can't I?"*
  - o   *"She sleeps around with everyone else; it's my turn."*
  - o   *"We have already been messing around; she has no right to be such a 'cocktease.'"*
- **Dangerous world:** *The belief that you live in a "dog-eat-dog world" and if you don't act on your desires, someone will "beat you to it."*

Group Discussion:

The main idea here is to understand how sex-specific thinking errors have developed as a result of an unhealthy sexual framework. When an individual has developed an unhealthy sexual framework through which they see the world and others, and their personal experiences support those beliefs, the beliefs are reinforced. This makes it much more likely that someone will commit a sexual offense.[3]

Skills Trainer: You will now explain the difference between stable dynamic and stable acute risk factors:

Over the last few decades, researchers have studied what factors make it more likely that a person will reoffend.[4] While static risk factors increase an individual's risk of reoffending, these factors do not change, because they are fixed factors. For example, a person cannot change their age, the characteristics of their victim(s), or the length of their criminal record. However, dynamic risk factors—or risk factors that can change—are what we target in treatment. You may notice that these risk factors occur at the "ongoing triggers" or "treading water" phase of your offense staircase (see Handout 8.1: My Offense Staircase).

There are also risk factors that are important to pay attention to during the "immediate triggers" phase of the offense staircase. Review Handout 7.2: Risk Factors for Reoffending, and put a checkmark next to your general risk factors, and a star next to your risk factors that arise or get stronger immediately before you offend.

For an example of common risk factors that arise prior to offending, see Handout 7.5: Identifying Immediate Situations that Could Lead to Relapse.

In addition to identifying risk factors, we want clients to address their protective factors, or factors that help minimize risk.[5] Working from a strengths-based perspective includes helping clients recognize factors and apply them in their daily lives. Protective factors are also dynamic, as they can change throughout the course of treatment. Carefully review Handout 7.3: Protective Factors, so participants understand each factor and can identify their specific risk and protective factors for the homework (Handout 7.4).

Handout 7.1: Thinking Errors

Self-talk (automatic thoughts):

- What we say to ourselves about ourselves, others, the world; our inner dialog.

Thinking errors are likely present when:

- You experience unusually intense emotions.
- Intense emotions last an unusually long period of time.
- You feel a very strong emotion that most people in the same situation would not feel to that extent.
- Your emotional state contributes to behavior that is harmful to yourself or others.

Types of thinking errors:

- **"But" statements:** Making an excuse and then qualifying it, or negating a rational statement.
  - Example: "I didn't practice my skills or do my homework this week, but I have been really busy at work."
  - Example: "I really like coming to group, but I just don't have time to practice my skills during the week."
- **"Mental filters" (can be overly positive or overly negative):** Thinking that things are the way you want to see them, rather than how they really are.
  - <u>Positive filter</u>: Being overly positive/optimistic even when things are not going well.
    - Example: "She is acting disinterested, but I know she is just playing hard to get."

- Negative filter: Ignoring the positives and only focusing on the negatives about yourself, others, or situations.
  - Example: "She does not want to have sex with me tonight. Here we go again. I am such a loser, and no one wants me."
- Causes problems because:
  - It promotes unrealistic thinking.
  - You do not try to change because you are convinced you are right (either way).
- **"Mind reading":** Acting as if you can tell what other people are thinking, feeling, doing, or going to do without asking them first. You make assumptions.
  - Example: You are at a party and someone walks in and smiles at you. You assume they are interested in you, and do not consider that they could just be polite.
  - Example: A woman wears a short skirt and low-cut blouse, and you assume that she is trying to get your or other men's attention.
  - Example: Your friend cancels evening plans with you, and you assume that they are blowing you off for something/someone better.
  - Causes problems because:
    - You assume what you want to assume without awareness of others and without checking with them.
    - You expect others to "read your mind" and act the way you want them to act.
    - You do not get your needs met and/or have strong reactions when people do not "read your mind"/know what you're thinking or feeling, or what you want.
- **"Fortune telling" (positive or negative):** Thinking you can predict the future and "know" that something will turn out positively or negatively without real evidence.
  - Positive fortune telling: Telling yourself that everything will work out well, with no strong evidence.
    - Example: "She's talking to me and smiling. She clearly wants to have sex with me."
  - Causes problems because:
    - It can set you up for a big crash/major disappointment.
  - Negative fortune telling: You tell yourself that everything will turn out badly without strong evidence.

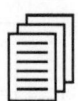

- Example: You see an attractive person and think, "I'm not going to bother talking to them because they will think I'm fat and unattractive."
- Causes problems because:
  - You justify not taking risks in relationships or in life out of fear.
- **"All-or-nothing" (or "black-and-white") thinking":** Thinking of life in extremes; rigid thinking. You (or others) are either a total failure or perfect; something is either right or wrong.
- Example: "I know she's underage and it's wrong, but I've already started driving to meet her, so I might as well just go."
- Example: You are masturbating and a thought of your victim pops into your head. You continue to masturbate because you are already close to orgasm.
- Causes problems because:
  - You avoid the fact that there is more than one way to do, think, or feel about something.
  - You do not respect others' views and cannot negotiate conflict.
- **Labeling:** Attaching negative labels to yourself, others, and/or the world. You may take one behavior or situation and apply a label to describe a whole person.
- Example: Your friend gets out of a relationship and into a new one within a few days. You think, "They're such a slut."
- Example: Your probation officer says something that upsets you and you say, "My P.O is an asshole."
- Causes problems because:
  - You push people away and do not give them the benefit of the doubt.
  - You think you know/understand people better than you do.
  - It negatively impacts relationships because people think you are judging them.
- **"Should" statements:** You try to motivate yourself by thinking, "I should do this," or "I shouldn't do that" (using judgmental words).
  - Examples: After you did a thorough job completing an assignment, your therapist provides you with a critique you do not like. You think, "I should have worked harder. I should have known better …"
  - Causes problems because:
    - You lose touch with what you have done, and with what you enjoy/like/want to do.
    - You lose sight of seeing things as being a choice (e.g. "It's natural for men to be attracted to children").

- You judge others ("They shouldn't have …").
- You set up a power struggle with yourself.
- **Control and manipulation:** You focus on getting other people to think, feel, or do things differently (the way you prefer); you may be "nice" in order to get what you want.
  - Example: "I tutor that kid two days per week so that I can spend more time with him and get him to trust me. Once I know he trusts me, I can touch him wherever I want."
  - Causes problems because:
    - It can feel good in the short term, or make you feel powerful or important, but it will lead others to dislike/distrust you in the long term.
    - People often pick up on this type of behavior and will avoid you.
    - Your relationships are based on fear or superficialities, not on respect.
  - **Victim stance ("poor me"):** Viewing oneself as a victim and blaming others for one's problems.
  - Example: You're in a fight with your partner and you hit them. You say, "It was their fault I hit them. They shouldn't have spoken to me that way."
  - Example: "She sleeps with everyone, but she called the police on me when I tried to have sex with her."
  - Causes problems because:
    - You do not take responsibility for your own actions. Everything is someone else's fault.
    - You tell people that they "make" you feel a certain way instead of taking ownership of your feelings.
    - You are often angry or resentful of people.
    - You feel justified to act out against others or blame others because you believe they have set you up somehow.
    - You ruin your relationships because people do not want to interact with those who cannot take responsibility; you are perceived as "whiny" or "obnoxious."
- **Self-focused:** Having an overly positive view of oneself; lacking empathy for others; thinking one is better than others ("above the rules"); not believing there should be consequences for one's actions; believing one has done nothing wrong.
  - Examples: You have been in three serious long-term relationships, but your partners have all left you. You think, "I don't know what's wrong with them. I didn't do anything to push them away."

- Causes problems because:
  - You are prone to telling yourself that you have the answers and do not need to listen to/do what others are telling or asking of you.
  - You become overly focused on your own thoughts, feelings, and experiences, and do not pay attention to others around you.
  - It negatively impacts relationships because people find you self-absorbed.

Homework: My sexual thinking errors

For this assignment:

- List your sexual thinking errors.
- Briefly describe a time you had each thinking error.
- Explain why it was a thinking error.

If you need more space, please use the back of the page.

Thinking errors	An example from my life	Why it is a thinking error
1.		
2.		
3.		
4.		
5.		
6.		

Handout 7.2: Risk Factors for Reoffending

What is risk?

A prediction of the likelihood of reoffending

Static risk factors

Factors that cannot change through treatment.

- Age (the younger the individual, the higher their risk).
- Criminal history (a longer history of crimes and the presence of violent offenses indicate higher risk).
- Victim's age/sex (people who offend against young males and strangers have higher risk).
- Deviant sexual preferences/arousal (see below).

Dynamic risk factors

Factors that *can* change through treatment. These are what we will focus on!

- **Problems with sexual self-regulation (e.g., deviant sexual interests, sexual preoccupation, using sex to cope):**
  - Deviant sexual interests (e.g., engaging in sexual acts with non-consenting people; this includes sex with minors).
    - *Why?* People who are attracted to engaging in illegal sexual behaviors are more likely to seek out the individuals or situations that excite them, which triggers them to act on this attraction.
  - Sexual preoccupation
    - *Why?* People who are sexually preoccupied think about sex too much. They oversexualize people and situations. They may place themselves in situations where there is an increased likelihood of offending.

- Using sex to cope
  - *Why?* General lack of self-control; problems controlling sexual impulses; using sex to cope with feelings; overvaluing sex in the pursuit of happiness.
- **Problems with general self-regulation (e.g., hostility/negative emotionality, poor problem solving, impulsiveness, employment instability, substance abuse, intoxication during the offense, hostility/anger):**
  - *Why?* An unstable lifestyle that involves manipulating, exploiting, or violating the rights of others. This includes rule breaking, poor employment, and impulsive behavior. Uncooperative with supervision.
- **Negative social influences:**
  - *Why?* People who engage in illegal activities are more likely to do so if their friends do, too. For example, your friends may be tolerant of inappropriate sexual behavior, talk about sex frequently, or objectify or sexualize others.
- **Intimacy deficits (e.g., emotional identification with minors, inability to establish a stable relationship, hostility toward women, general social rejection/loneliness, lack of concern for others):**
  - Emotional identification with minors:
    - *Why?* People who emotionally identify with children are at increased risk of placing themselves in situations where they have more access to children in order to actively pursue connections with children. In addition, people with intimacy deficits have trouble relating to adults in a healthy/respectful way.
  - Inability to establish a stable relationship:
    - *Why?* People who lack positive social supports are more likely to experience negative moods and loneliness, which may increase the likelihood of using sex to cope.
  - Hostility/anger toward women:
    - *Why?* Related to impulsivity and antisocial behavior, objectification/oversexualizing women; the belief that the individual is being victimized by women, or that women exist to serve men's needs/desires.
  - Lack of concern for others:
    - *Why?* When people do not have regard for the feelings or experiences of others, they are more likely to have trouble finding and/or maintaining a healthy, stable relationship.
  - Uncooperative with supervision:
    - *Why?* People who do not follow the rules of supervision tend to be more impulsive and have interpersonal problems.

Handout 7.3: Protective Factors

Factors that people either have or may be able to develop that minimize their risk of reoffending include the following:

- **Empathy** vs. blaming others or taking a victim stance.
- **Appropriate problem-solving and emotion regulation skills** vs. allowing yourself to indulge in compulsive thoughts and behavior.
- **Self-control and emotion management** vs. impulsive actions.
- **Recognition and respect of the rights of others** (e.g., women are not objects who owe you anything; not harming others) vs. hostility toward women and others.
- **Acceptance and management of your sexuality** (e.g., avoiding children, seeking and having relationships with consenting adults, not masturbating to thoughts of illegal behavior, not using sex/masturbation to cope with negative feelings) vs. ignoring or trying to change your sexuality, using sex to cope, masturbating to thoughts of illegal behavior.
- **Openness to treatment, support, and supervision** (e.g., medication compliance, positive attitude toward treatment, acceptance of support, managing your risk, accepting the rules even if you do not like them) vs. lack of cooperation or negative attitude.
- **Self-care** (e.g., eating healthy foods, exercising, avoiding drugs, spending time with positive social influences, finding time for activities you enjoy) vs. isolation; not maintaining physical health, or participating in enjoyable activities.
- **Intimacy** (e.g., effective communication with others, seeking an emotional connection with others, trust, effectively deciding when to "let things go") vs. identification with children, or getting stuck in harmful relationship patterns (see Handout 12.1: The Four Horsemen).
- **Stable employment, housing, and finances.**

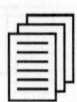

Handout 7.4: My Personal Risk and Protective Factors

1. _____

    Why this a risk factor for me:

    _____

    _____

    _____

    An example from my life is:

    _____

    _____

    I can decrease this risk by [insert skill(s)]:

    _____

    _____

    _____

2. _____

    Why this is a risk factor for me:

    _____

    _____

    _____

    An example from my life is:

    _____

    _____

    _____

I can decrease this risk by:

_____

_____

_____

3. _____

_____

_____

_____

Why this is a risk factor for me:

_____

_____

_____

An example from my life is:

_____

_____

_____

I can decrease this risk by:

_____

_____

_____

4. _____

Why this is a risk factor for me:

_____

_____

_____

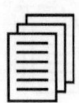

An example from my life is:

_____

_____

_____

I can decrease this risk by:

_____

_____

_____

5. _____

Why this is a risk factor for me:

_____

_____

_____

An example from my life is:

_____

_____

_____

I can decrease this risk by:

_____

_____

_____

6. _____

Why this is a risk factor for me:

_____

_____

_____

An example from my life is:

_____

_____

_____

I can decrease this risk by:

_____

_____

_____

7. _____

Why this is a risk factor for me:

_____

_____

_____

An example from my life is:

_____

_____

_____

I can decrease my risk by:

_____

_____

_____

My protective factors

_____

_____

_____

_____

_____

_____

_____

_____

_____

_____

_____

_____

_____

_____

Handout 7.5: Identifying Immediate Situations that Could Lead to Relapse[6]

- **Access to a victim or potential victim:** Placing yourself in situation where minors are present; grooming behaviors.
- **Hostility:** An increase in anger or significant frustration; distress; blaming others.
- **Sexual preoccupation**: An increase in masturbation; fantasizing about illegal behavior; having sex with multiple partners; making frequent sexual comments/innuendos.
- **Rejection of supervision:** Not following the conditions of your probation/parole.
- **Emotional collapse:** Allowing problems to spiral out of control; intrusive thoughts; compulsive behavior; not using effective or healthy coping skills to address problems.
- **Change in social supports:** The death of a loved one; rejection from a partner, family, or friend; problems at work.
- **Substance use:** Using drugs or alcohol after a period of abstinence; increasing substance use.

Notes

1 Ward & Keenan (1999, 124).
2 Polacheck & Ward (2002).
3 Ward (2000).
4 Hanson & Bussiere (1998).
5 Association for the Treatment and Prevention of Sexual Abuse guidelines (2014, sec. 5.09) state that clinicians should:

> explore and document a client's strengths, assets, and protective factors which may include but are not limited to the following areas:
> - Prosocial Community supports and influences, and others involved in care and treatment;
> - Structure and support that promote maintaining success (e.g., limited access to potential victims;
> - Healthy, age appropriate, normative, long-term intimate and sexual relationships;
> - Motivation to change;
> - Insight, understanding, and management of risk factors;
> - Appropriate problem solving and emotional management skills; and
> - Employment, financial, and residential stability.

6 Brankley, Helmus, & Hanson (2017).

References

Association for the Treatment of Sexual Abusers. (2014). *Practice Guidelines for the Assessment, Treatment, and Management of Male Adult Sexual Abusers.*

Brankley A. E., Helmus L.-M., Hanson R. K. (2017). *STABLE-2007 evaluator workbook: Updated recidivism rates (includes combinations with Static-99R, Static-2002R, and Risk Matrix 2000).* Unpublished report. Ottawa, ON: Public Safety Canada.

Hanson R. K., & Bussière M. T. (1998). Predicting relapse: A meta-analysis of sexual offender recidivism studies. *Journal of Consulting and Clinical Psychology, 66*(2), 348–362. https://doi.org/10.1037/0022-006X.66.2.348

Polaschek D. L. L., & Ward, T. (2002). The implicit theories of potential rapists: What our questionnaires tell us. *Aggression and Violent Behavior, 7,* 385–406. https://doi.org/10.1016/S1359-1789(01)00063-5

Ward T. (2000). Sexual offenders' cognitive distortions as implicit theories. *Aggression and Violent Behavior, 5*(5), 491–507. https://doi.org/10.1016/S1359-1789(98)00036-6

Ward T., & Keenan T. (1999). Child molesters' implicit theories. *Journal of Interpersonal Violence, 14*(8), 821–838. https://doi.org/10.1177/088626099014008003

Understanding My Offence

8

When reviewing Handout 7.2: My Risk Factors for Reoffending, make sure to provide participants with feedback if they have missed a risk factor that is specifically relevant to their offense behavior. I have found that clients sometimes have difficulty understanding how certain risk factors relate to them, so this will be important to address in the group.

Despite understanding their risk factors, clients still may be unclear about how to recognize when they are placing themselves in risky situations. Acute risk factors, once again, are factors that change in the short term and are important for clients to be able to identify because they have the potential to lead to reoffending. Review Handout 7.5: Identifying Immediate Situations that Could Lead to Relapse, and explain that these are considered "crisis situations." Explain to clients that if they are experiencing acute risk factors, they should reach out to their individual therapist right away.

Group Activity: Ask clients to break up into groups of three, and create a list of alternative statements, or challenges to their sexual thinking errors. For example: "If the barista is talking to me at the coffee shop, she wants to have sex with me." An alternative statement might be: "She may be talking to me because it is her job to be friendly to customers." After 10–15 minutes, ask the group to come back together and share their alternative statements to each sexual thinking error. (It is helpful if one of the skills trainers takes notes and writes down all group members' ideas and creates a typed document to provide the following week.) Once you have completed the exercise, ask clients what they notice about the lists they have generated. The main point of this exercise

DOI: 10.4324/9781003451099-11

is for clients to acknowledge that many of the sexual thinking errors are statements they commonly hear from others who have not been convicted of a sex offense, or that have been normalized by society; and for them to develop alternative, effective and legal responses to these thinking errors.

Skills Trainer: Now, move on to Handout 8.1: My Offense Staircase. Explain that there is a unique pathway each person followed that led to their offense(s). The offense staircase is similar to a behavior chain analysis, but with additional factors leading up to the offense and what happened after the offense. Moreover, it encourages clients to carefully reevaluate their offense now they have gained more skills and thus have a better understanding of the many factors involved in their offending. Carefully review each step and provide examples. You may want to use the example of John Doe to help participants better understand the model. The homework assignment this week will focus on participants addressing their individual pathways to offending.

While the offense staircase requires sequential thinking, some of your clients may be more abstract thinkers. In this case, let clients know that they can choose between Handout 8.1: My Offense Staircase and Handout 8.2: My Offense Volcano. Participants will complete Handout 8.3 over the next week to gain a more nuanced understanding of their own offense(s).

Example:

- **Stability:** When John's life is stable, he is working full time, only drinking socially, and not feeling overwhelmed by constant depression, anxiety, or anger; and he and his wife are not fighting.

- **Ongoing triggers:** John has a history of depression, anxiety, and anger outbursts; but they come and go. He has a history of drinking heavily when he feels anxious and depressed.

- **Treading water:** John lost his job due to company downsizing, and he and his wife have started arguing about finances. He begins to feel depressed and anxious because he cannot support his family at the moment.

- **Immediate triggers:** John got into a fight with his wife and left the house to go to the bar, where he proceeded to get drunk.

- **Offence:** John left the bar with a woman he did not know. He went to her house, and they began to make out. He took off his pants and she said, "I don't want to have sex." John said, "Why would you bring me back to your home and make out with me if you didn't want to have sex? You're leading me on." John proceeded to have sex with the woman against her will.

- **Post-offense:** John left the woman's house and went home. He forgot about what happened until the police came to his house two days later. The woman had called the police to report the rape. At the police station, John maintained that the sex was consensual.

Handout 8.1: My Offense Staircase

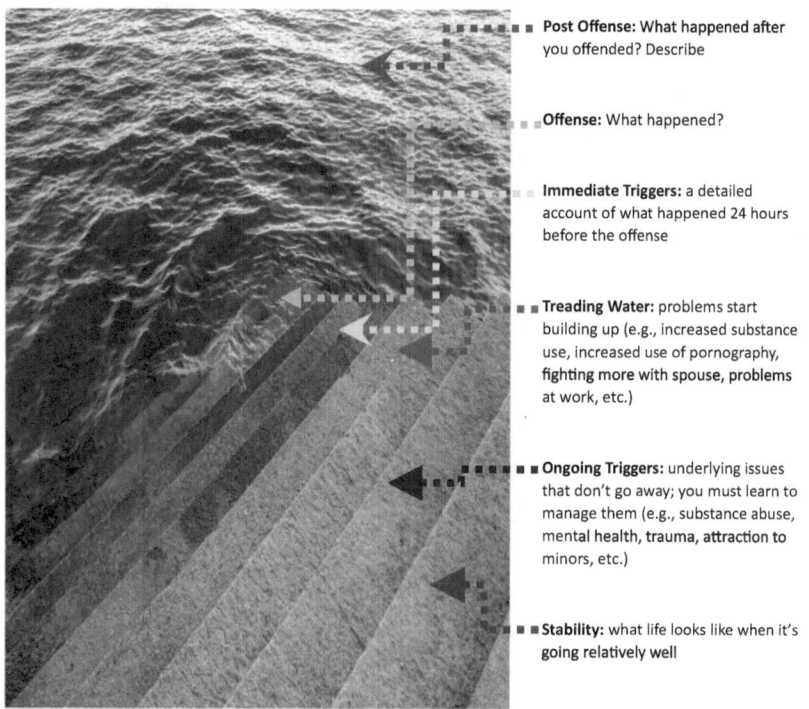

Post Offense: What happened after you offended? Describe

Offense: What happened?

Immediate Triggers: a detailed account of what happened 24 hours before the offense

Treading Water: problems start building up (e.g., increased substance use, increased use of pornography, fighting more with spouse, problems at work, etc.)

Ongoing Triggers: underlying issues that don't go away; you must learn to manage them (e.g., substance abuse, mental health, trauma, attraction to minors, etc.)

Stability: what life looks like when it's going relatively well

Image 8.1 Staircase descending into the water

Handout 8.2: My Offense Volcano

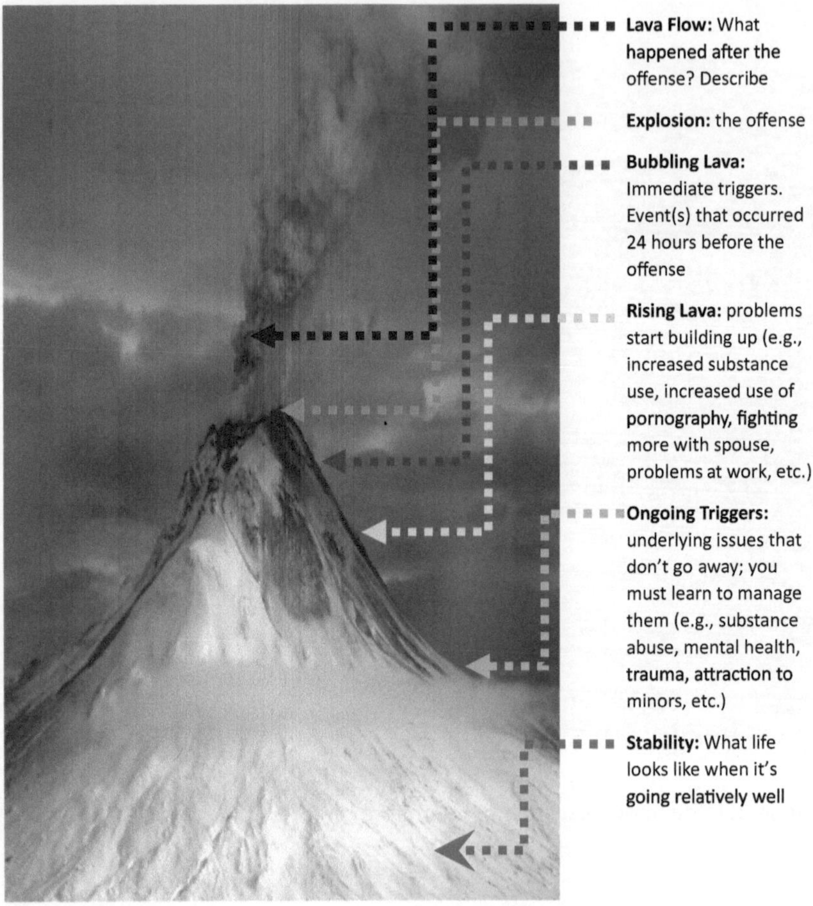

Lava Flow: What happened after the offense? Describe

Explosion: the offense

Bubbling Lava: Immediate triggers. Event(s) that occurred 24 hours before the offense

Rising Lava: problems start building up (e.g., increased substance use, increased use of pornography, fighting more with spouse, problems at work, etc.)

Ongoing Triggers: underlying issues that don't go away; you must learn to manage them (e.g., substance abuse, mental health, trauma, attraction to minors, etc.)

Stability: What life looks like when it's going relatively well

Image 8.2 Volcano

Handout 8.3: My Offence Staircase or Offense Volcano

For this homework assignment, you will complete your personal offense staircase or offense volcano (your choice).

Stability

What does your life look like when it is going well?

_____

_____

_____

_____

_____

_____

Some of my general thinking errors are:

_____

_____

_____

_____

_____

_____

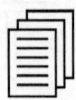

Ongoing triggers

What are some underlying issues or problems you struggle with when life is going well?

_____

_____

_____

_____

_____

_____

Which of these issues could put you at risk of offending again? Explain.

_____

_____

_____

_____

_____

_____

Treading water/rising lava

Describe what happened or changed in each of these areas of your life that led you to "tread water."

My physical health:

_____

_____

_____

_____

_____

My thoughts/self-talk:

_____

_____

_____

_____

_____

_____

My money management:

_____

_____

_____

_____

_____

_____

My attitudes, values, and beliefs:

_____

_____

_____

_____

_____

_____

My spiritual involvement:

_____

_____

_____

_____

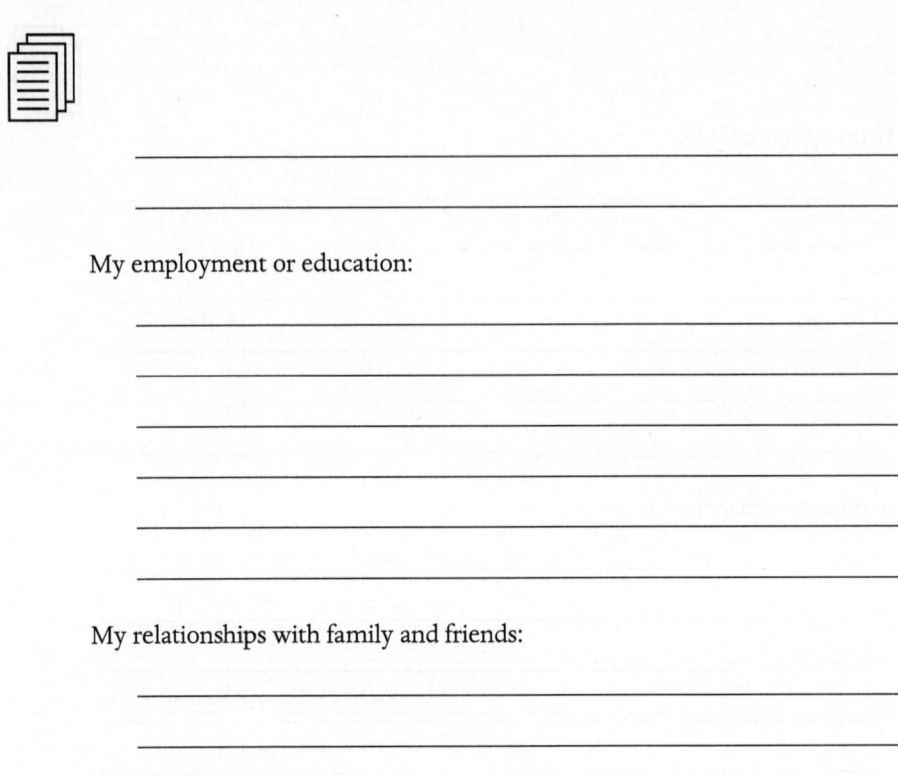

_____

_____

My employment or education:

_____

_____

_____

_____

_____

My relationships with family and friends:

_____

_____

_____

_____

_____

_____

My substance use or abuse:

_____

_____

_____

_____

_____

_____

The way I spend my leisure time / recreational activities:

_____

_____

_____

_____

_____

_____

My sexual behavior:

_____

_____

_____

_____

_____

My fantasies and arousal patterns:

_____

_____

_____

_____

_____

My use of pornography:

_____

_____

_____

_____

_____

Other life stressors:

_____

_____

_____

_____

_____

_____

Other people have noticed the following changes in my behavior:

_____

_____

_____

_____

_____

_____

My thinking errors during this time were:

_____

_____

_____

_____

_____

_____

Immediate triggers/bubbling lava:

How did you form a relationship with the victim(s)?

_____

_____

_____

_____

_____

_____

What did you do, specifically, to create an opportunity for offending?

_____

_____

_____

_____

_____

_____

What steps did you take to plan your offense (i.e., what made you excited to offend)?

_____

_____

_____

_____

_____

My thinking errors at this time included:

_____

_____

_____

_____

_____

_____

The offense/explosion

My offense involved the following behaviors:

_____

_____

_____

_____

_____

_____

These were my thinking errors while I was committing my offense:

_____

_____

_____

_____

_____

Post-offense/lava flow:

This is what happened immediately following the offense (include the behaviors and actions of both the victim and you):

_____

_____

_____

_____

_____

This is what happened the day after the offense (include the behaviors and actions of both the victim and you):

_____

_____

_____

_____

_____

_____

This is what happened within a few weeks of the offense:

_____

_____

_____

_____

_____

These were my thinking errors after I committed the offense:

_____

_____

_____

_____

_____

This is what my life looks like right now:

_____

_____

_____

_____

_____

_____

These are the behaviors I need to be aware of to avoid future offending:

_____

_____

_____

_____

_____

_____

Part III

Interpersonal Effectiveness Skills

Intimacy, Relationships, and Interpersonal Myths

9

Skills Trainer: As previously discussed, many men convicted of a sexual offense have experienced invalidating relationships at some point in their lives. This invalidation can lead to distrust of others, anger toward others, and an inability to recognize verbal and non-verbal cues from others. We cannot ignore a history of trauma for a significant proportion of sex offenders.[1] By using the biopsychosocial perspective, we can better understand higher rates of adverse childhood experiences and how they may play a role in sexual offending. Briefly explain this and provide examples of how biological, psychological, and social factors converge and help us better understand how poor relationships are implicated in sexual offending (you can refer back to Chapter 3).

Once again, briefly explain and provide examples of how biological, psychological, and social factors converge, and how they help clients better understand how problematic relationships, or a lack of relationships, is implicated in sexual offending. Remember that a history of trauma is not a causal factor for sex offending; however, there is a strong correlation.[2]

Ask clients to fill out Handout 9.1: My Interpersonal Skills Rating Scale. Once they have completed it, go around the room and ask them what they noticed.

Why Are Interpersonal Effectiveness Skills Important?

Skills Trainer:
Research shows that people who have positive interactions with others tend to experience less stress, depression, and anxiety, and improved cognitive skills.[3]

DOI: 10.4324/9781003451099-13

Interpersonal effectiveness skills are necessary in order to lead a more fulfilling life. We have to be mindful of the various factors and behaviors that increase intimacy. Intimacy is not only sexual. You can think of it as "emotional closeness" to another person.

Group Discussion: Ask group members to list various factors and behaviors that contribute to intimacy. Write them down on the whiteboard.

Skills Trainer: If clients have not addressed certain factors and behaviors, make sure you list the following too:[4]

- Effective, open communication with others.
- Spending quality time together.
- Sharing positive experiences with others.
- How to interact effectively with others.
- Demonstrating respect.
- Trust.
- Shared goals and values.
- Liking things other than sex or physical appearance about the other person.

Skills Trainer:
There are many myths about interpersonal relationships—whether with a sexual partner, or with friends and family. The following myths may stem from feelings of low self-worth or beliefs of superiority. All of these beliefs get in the way of having effective, healthy relationships because they alienate others or make them uncomfortable.

Review Handout 9.2: Interpersonal Myths and explain how each belief tends to make others uncomfortable. Ask clients to check the circle that corresponds to their beliefs about interpersonal relationships.

There are three main goals of learning interpersonal effectiveness skills:

- *Obtaining what one wants from a relationship while maintaining self-respect.*
- *Developing and maintaining relationships.*
- *"Walking the middle path," or finding balance within one's relationships. This means that both or all individuals involved in the relationship are in equilibrium. You can think about this as like two people on a seesaw. The purpose of a seesaw is to teach people how to make physical adjustments so that their weight is evenly distributed, and the seesaw is parallel.*

One major risk factor for sexual reoffending concerns problems related to intimacy. These can result from the individual trying too hard to please others and thus ignoring his own needs; or from not being in tune with others' needs. Whether these men overidentify with children, harbor anger toward women, lose attraction to their partner, or tend to isolate, men who have committed a sexual offense often have significant problems with their interpersonal relationships. This problem is often compounded when they have experienced trauma in their life.

Ask participants to look at Handout 9.3: Passive, Aggressive, and Assertiveness Defined.

Being effective in your interpersonal relationships means that you are able to negotiate with others—without being manipulative—in order to have your needs met, and to do it without compromising your own values, goals, or integrity.

As discussed previously, oftentimes people react rather than respond to a frustrating situation or interaction (emotional mind). This means that people may either "give in" without considering their personal boundaries (passivity); "explode," thereby violating others' boundaries (aggression); or do a little of both (passive-aggression).

For example, your partner wants to take a walk in the park, but this is a violation of your terms of probation or parole. Your partner is angry and says, "If you hadn't committed that offense, we could do more things together."

- *Passivity: Not saying anything; looking at the floor; saying, "You're right. I've ruined our lives."*
- *Aggression: Yelling or swearing at your partner; calling them names; erupting in anger. "I know that! Do you think I'm dumb or something? Get off my back for once!"*
- *Passive-aggression: You make a snarky comment such as, "I know. Everything is always my fault," and walk away.*

All of these responses are problematic because you are not demonstrating respect for yourself, for the other person, or for both parties. In order to move beyond these unhelpful responses, there must be a middle ground, or balance. This synthesis is referred to as "assertiveness." When you are assertive, you acknowledge your feelings and those of the other person. Assertiveness involves responding to the other person and the situation, rather than reacting. The difference between responding and reacting is that a response is thoughtful and non-judgmental, and is more likely to de-escalate a potentially problematic situation. Reactions, on the other hand, are immediate expressions of emotions (i.e., you have not stopped to think about how to respond to the other person). Reactions can result in the other person becoming defensive, and the situation escalating. Let's consider the example I just gave you. Instead of reacting to your partner, you respond by saying, "I know that this is one of the consequences of my offense, and I would really like to take a walk in the park with you. I know that what I did affects your life, too, but it hurts me that you keep bringing it up." In this scenario, you acknowledge your partner's feelings and experiences, and your own, without yelling or insulting your partner. Moreover, you stand up for yourself and demonstrate self-respect.

Group Discussion: Ask clients to consider a time when they responded to a situation unskillfully (i.e., passively, aggressively, or passive-aggressively). Have each client practice describing the situation neutrally ("Only use the facts!"), how they interpreted the situation, and how they could have responded differently. Be sure to elicit group feedback.

Practice Exercise: Ask clients to break up into pairs. Client A will make the requests listed below to Client B. Client B will practice assertive responses. Next, the clients will switch places, so Client A has an opportunity to practice his responses too. The skills trainer will walk around the room and listen to one or more of each pair's responses. If their response is appropriate and effective, say, "That sounds good! How come that was an effective response?" If their response does not sound appropriate or effective, ask, "How do you see this response as effective? Is there a way that your response could be more effective?"

Examples of scenarios/requests:

- For individuals who have substance misuse problems or are not allowed to drink as part of their probation/parole conditions: "Come have a couple drinks with me at the bar."
- For individuals who are attracted to minors: "Come over to my place and hang out. My kids will be upstairs."
- At a party: "That chick over there is hot and she's checking you out. Take her upstairs and have sex with her."
- For individuals who frequently "drop everything" to help others: "I know you've been super busy all week, but I really need you to help me move this weekend."

Handout 9.1: My Interpersonal Skills Rating Scale

Place a checkmark in the box that best corresponds to your effectiveness using each skill.

	1. Extremely ineffective	2. Somewhat effective	3. Moderately effective	4. Somewhat effective	5. Extremely effective
Saying "no" when you do not want to do something					
Asking for help					
Sharing your feelings and thoughts					
Lashing out when upset (physically or verbally)					
Being non-judgmental					
Apologizing when you are wrong					
Actively listening to others (e.g., eye contact, not interrupting)					
Getting defensive/ angry					
Other?					

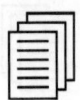

Handout 9.2: Interpersonal Myths

These are common myths among individuals who feel badly about themselves:

- I am not worthy of having healthy, happy relationships.
- I am a bad person.
- No one will want to date me because I am a registered sex offender.
- I don't have the right to speak up; I should "know my place."
- I should like everyone.
- I don't need to have relationships. I am happy being a loner.

These are common myths among individuals who feel superiority in their interactions:

- Other people should know what I want/need without me having to tell them.
- I am just a good guy who is constantly misunderstood.
- I am unique/special and people should realize that.
- I am the victim in all of this.
- You can't trust anyone because they will always burn you in the end.
- Only "soft" men express their emotions to others.
- I don't need to work at having or improving my relationships.
- I have the right to do and say whatever I want.
- Everyone should like me.

Handout 9.3: Passive, Aggressive, and Assertive Defined

Passive:	Aggressive:	Passive-Aggressive:	Assertive:
Low self-esteem; desires acceptance; frequently feels shame or guilt; has poor boundaries; feels powerless.	Overly/ inappropriately direct; own needs come first; inflated sense of self; hostile; desires power.	Indirect and dishonest about thoughts and feelings; harbors anger but does not communicate it; says or does something in a sneaky way to "get back" at the other person.	Clearly defined boundaries; clearly and calmly communicates thoughts and feelings without blaming others.
Example: Simon feels aroused but does not communicate this with his partner because he is afraid of being turned down.	**Example:** Simon feels aroused so he pulls his partner's pants down and forces himself on them.	**Example:** Simon feels aroused and asks his partner to have sex. The partner says they are not in the mood, so Simon gives her the silent treatment for the rest of the day. He thinks to himself, 'I'll show *them*!'	**Example:** Simon feels aroused ask asks his partner to have sex. His partner is not in the mood, so Simon says, "Okay, let me know when you are," or "I've noticed that it has been a while since we have had sex and I'm feeling bad about it. How can we address this issue together?"

Notes

1 For example, Reavis, Looman, Franco, and Rojas (2013) found that sexual offenders report higher scores on the adverse childhood experiences scale—specifically related to physical, emotional, and sexual abuse—than the general population. Additionally, studies show that between approximately 26% (Reavis et al., 2013) and 38% of all sexual offenders have a history of being sexually abused (Levenson, Willis, & Prescott, 2017); and that sexual offenders are over times more likely to experience sexual abuse than non-sexual offenders (Jespersen, Lalumiere, & Seto, 2009).
2 Levenson, Willis, & Prescot (2016).
3 Coutinho, Silva, & Decety (2014).
4 Frei & Shaver (2002); Gottman (1993); Reis et al. (2010).

References

Coutinho, J. F., Silva, P. O., & Decety, J. (2014). Neurosciences, empathy, and healthy interpersonal relationships: recent findings and implications for counseling psychology. *Journal of Counseling Psychology, 61*(4), 541. https://doi.org/10.1037/cou0000021

Frei, J. R., & Shaver, P. R. (2002). Respect in close relationships: Prototype definition, self-report assessment, and initial correlates. *Personal Relationships, 9*(2), 121–139. https://doi.org/10.1111/1475-6811.00008

Levenson, J. S., Willis, G. M., & Prescott, D. S. (2016). Adverse childhood experiences in the lives of male sex offenders: Implications for trauma-informed care. *Sexual Abuse, 28*(4), 340–359. https://doi.org/10.1177/1079063214535819

Gottman, J. M. (1993). The roles of conflict engagement, escalation, and avoidance in marital interaction: A longitudinal view of five types of couples. *Journal of Consulting and Clinical Psychology, 61*(1), 6–15. https://doi.org/10.1037//0022-006X.61.1.6

Jespersen, A. F., Lalumière, M. L., & Seto, M. C. (2009). Sexual abuse history among adult sex offenders and non-sex offenders: A meta-analysis. *Child Abuse & Neglect, 33*(3), 179–192. https://doi.org/10.1016/j.chiabu.2008.07.004

Reavis, J. A., Looman, J., Franco, K. A., & Rojas, B. (2013). Adverse childhood experiences and adult criminality: How long must we live before we possess our own lives? *The Permanente Journal, 17*(2), 44–48. https://doi.org/10.7812/TPP/12-072

Reis, H., Smith, S. M., Carmichael, C. L., Caprariello, P. A., Tsai, F. F., Rodrigues, A., & Maniaci, M. R. (2010). Are you happy for me? How sharing positive events with others provides personal and interpersonal benefits. *Journal of Personality and Social Psychology, 99*(2), 311–329. https://doi.org/10.1037/a0018344

Mindful Communication and Boundary Violations

10

DOI: 10.4324/9781003451099-14

Skills Trainer: Ask participants to take out Handout 10.1: Mindful Communication.

Many people have difficulty expressing their thoughts or feelings, asking for what they need, and setting boundaries (e.g., trouble saying "no"). These difficulties often stem from a person's desire to be "liked," or to "fit in." There are a few ways that clients can be assertive rather than passive in these situations. The following are ways to be more effective in these situations, and questions to ask yourself prior to reacting to the situation:

- *Fact-checking: "Have I interpreted what the other person is saying or assumed they meant something, without asking for clarification?"*
- *Using wise mind: "Is my response non-judgmental, and focused specifically on the current interaction?"*
- *Developing a rational response: "Is my response effective? Have I acknowledged the other person's desires or needs while also acknowledging my own? Is my response logical and factual?"*
- *Practicing an opposite action: "Am I considering giving in to avoid problems? Do I feel like walking away?"*

Failure to use mindful communication can lead to boundary violations because it demonstrates a lack of awareness or sensitivity toward the other person. When you are not mindful in your communication with others, you may fail to recognize or respect the emotions or personal space of others. People who have committed sex crimes have violated the boundaries of others, and typically have trouble understanding and/or respecting other people's physical or emotional space. "Boundaries" can refer to physical space, such as standing an appropriate distance from someone when talking to them; or to an individual's right to maintain their psychological or emotional wellbeing.

In-group Assignment and Discussion: Review Handout 10.2: Boundary Violations with the group and ask them to place a checkmark next to the boundaries they have crossed. After doing this, participants should write an example of a time when they committed each checked boundary violation. After they have completed the worksheet (approximately 15–20 minutes), everyone will share two of the boundary violation scenarios they wrote down. Be sure to encourage the group to provide feedback to one another.

Explain that the homework this week will require group members to review the scenarios they wrote in Handout 10.3 and create a plan of action (Handout 10.4: My Plan of Action). The plan of action should list steps they will take to avoid violating someone's boundaries if they find themselves in a similar situation.

Handout 10.1: Mindful Communication

- Fact-checking: Have I interpreted what the other person is saying or assumed they meant something, without asking for clarification?
- Using wise mind: Is my response non-judgmental, and focused specifically on the current interaction?
- Developing a rational response: Is my response effective? Have I acknowledged the other person's desires or needs while also acknowledging my own? Is my response logical and factual?
- Practicing an opposite action: Am I considering giving in to avoid problems? Do I feel like walking away?

Handout 10.2: Boundary Violations

- Peeping.
- Exposing yourself.
- Frottage (rubbing against a non-consenting person).
- Placing yourself in a situation where minors will be / are present.
- Grooming behaviors.
- Touching someone without their permission.
- Standing too close to someone (perhaps they try to back up).
- Talking "at" someone (not allowing them the chance to speak).
- Asking too many personal questions.
- Oversharing personal information.
- Calling/texting too frequently (this is interpreted as being overly controlling or needy).
- Being overly sexual with/making sexual comments toward someone who is not your partner (this includes sexual jokes and commenting on their physique).
- Speaking over others.
- Overstaying your welcome.
- Frequently breaking promises.
- Constantly using someone as your emotional support without "giving back." This could also refer to frequently complaining to others.
- Asking someone why they are still single, or why they do not have children.
- Telling women to "smile."
- Trying to change another person.
- Being overly dependent on one person.
- Snooping in people's personal spaces, including phones and computers.
- Gaslighting (psychological manipulation where one person makes another person question their sanity, judgment, or perceptions; calling someone "crazy" or spreading rumors/gossip about them; making someone feel inadequate; lying about something you said or did).
- Isolating someone from their family/friends.
- "Love-bombing" (being overly affectionate and/or making grand romantic gestures at the beginning of a relationship).

- Not respecting another person's wishes (e.g., not giving them space; refusing to use a condom, or taking your condom off in the middle of sex without your partner's consent (this is also illegal); trying to change their mind).
- Viewing child pornography (also illegal).
- Other? _____

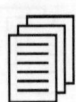

Handout 10.3: Times I Have Violated Someone's Boundaries

(If you need more space, use the back of the page)

1. _____
   _____
   _____
   _____
   _____
   _____
   _____

2. _____
   _____
   _____
   _____
   _____
   _____

3. _____
   _____
   _____
   _____
   _____
   _____

4. _____

_____

_____

_____

_____

_____

_____

_____

5. _____

_____

_____

_____

_____

_____

_____

Handout 10.4: My Plan of Action

List actions you can take (or not take) to avoid violating someone's boundaries if you are in a similar situation.

Situation #1:	
Situation #2:	
Situation #3:	
Situation #4:	
Situation #5	

DEAR MAN and GIVE FAST Skills

11

Skills Trainer:

People struggle with different aspects of being interpersonally effective. Many people do not feel comfortable asserting themselves by saying "no" to something they do not want to do. You may experience this difficulty too, or ignore the boundaries of others. As we discussed last week, sexual offenses are the result of individuals ignoring other people's boundaries. We have also learned that "no means no"; and that an absence of "yes" means "no." Let's say you are at a party where everyone is drinking. You have been flirting with another person all night and think that they want to go home with you to have sex. You ask them if they want to come over to your house. They say "no." What are some examples of inappropriate responses to this scenario? (E.g., swearing at the other person; calling them names; saying, "I don't care—I wasn't that into you anyway," or "I was just doing you a favor.")

What about if that person went to your house, did not want to have sex, but was too embarrassed to say "no"? They are willing to make out with you, but when you put your hand under their clothes, they push it away, sit up, or back away. These are non-verbal signals that are important to recognize. What would be the appropriate response in this situation?

Interpersonal effectiveness skills help you learn how to have appropriate interactions when something is not going the way you would like it to go. You can think about building and maintaining effective relationships like growing a plant. In order for plants to grow and stay alive, they must be nourished with proper soil, watered, and receive sunlight. In fact, scientists have learned that talking to your plants in a calm voice and playing music to them can help them

DOI: 10.4324/9781003451099-15

grow.[1] The idea here is that people, animals, and even plants thrive when they receive the "nourishment" they need.

Skills for building and maintaining effective interpersonal relationships can be remembered using the acronyms DEAR MAN (Handouts 11.1 and 11.2), and GIVE FAST. DEAR MAN can help you get what you want from an interaction without being manipulative. Consider this scenario: you think your partner is distancing themselves from you. You and your partner have stopped communicating; and when you do engage with each other, either your conversations are vague, or you end up arguing. You want to improve your relationship with your partner, but neither of you wants to make the first move by addressing the issue. When you encounter a frustrating or upsetting situation such as this, using your DEAR MAN skills can be helpful to express your needs and desires while respecting others' needs and desires, and to improve your communication with your partner (or anyone else).

Review Handout 11.1: DEAR MAN with the group and ask if they have questions.

Group Discussion: Use one of the examples above, or create another scenario. Clients will likely say that the example is easy, and that they have encountered much more difficult situations (which they likely have) in which employing these skills would be much harder, or perhaps even be perceived as impossible. Ask clients to volunteer and share an example of a situation where using these skills would have been more challenging, thus causing them to feel "stuck" about how to respond. Allow the group to come up with ways to use the skills in the client's situation.

DEAR MAN Skills

- **Describe the current interaction:** *When we feel frustrated by an interaction, we tend to react to others using our emotion mind. In a frustrating interaction, explain why you are feeling the way you do using only facts. (E.g., "I've noticed that we haven't been as close as we used to be.")*
- **Express thoughts or feelings about the interaction:** *(E.g., "I feel sad/badly that we haven't been communicating well.")*
- **Assert wishes in the situation:** *(E.g., "I would really like to improve our relationship, and I think sitting down and calmly talking about our issues would be helpful.")*
- **Reinforce:** *"Reinforcement" refers to rewarding the other person for doing what you want. You may need to address negative consequences here, too. (E.g., "I*

want to make things good again between us." If necessary, "Because I love you and want us both to be happy.") Reinforcement should also include verbal and/ or non-verbal communication after you get what you want. (E.g., smile, thank the person, give them a hug if they consent to it. Make sure they are aware that they have done something helpful, and that you are appreciative.)

- **_Mindful of needs:_** *Stay mindful of your boundaries, and those of others. Avoid distractions around you, or from the other person. Stick to the topic!*

- **_Appear confident:_** *You do not have to feel confident, but it is important to present yourself as such. For example, stand up straight, make good eye contact, and speak clearly and directly.*

- **_Negotiate:_** *Negotiation is not manipulation; it is a give-and-take solution to the problem. (E.g., your partner does not have time to talk right now. Let them know that you would like to talk when they have time. Ask if you can both agree on a good time to have the conversation.) Asking for a concrete day/time means that you are serious about having a conversation, yet also flexible.*

GIVE FAST Skills

- **_(Be) Gentle:_** *Being gentle during interactions is a means of being respectful. In other words, it means that you do not judge (e.g., "My partner is so needy that they can't let me go out for an hour with my friends), threaten (e.g., "You're just making me want leave and go back to hang out with them"), attack (e.g., "Why can't you ever cut me break? All you do is nag me!"), or completely dismiss what the other person is saying (e.g., walking away).*

- **_(Act) Interested:_** *This does not necessarily mean that you are interested in what the other person is saying, but rather that you act as though you are. When someone acts interested, they:*
  - *Actively listen to the other person's point of view.*
  - *Make eye contact with the other person (e.g., avoid looking down, around you, or at your phone).*
  - *Do not interrupt the other person; wait until they are done talking to respond.*

- **_Validate:_** *Validation is the recognition of another person's thoughts and feelings.*
  - *Consider how you might feel if you were in the other person's shoes.*
  - *Avoid taking a defensive stance.*
  - *Repeat what you heard the other person say (e.g., "I understand why you are upset with me. I should have called you to let you know I was going out with my friends").*

- *(Use an) Easy manner:* Put the other person at ease rather than being defensive, or having an attitude. You may want to touch your partner's hand and move closer with them to let them know you care about their feelings. You could also say something humorous to ease the tension (e.g., "This aging thing is no joke. I can't even remember what I had for breakfast this morning. I've got to do better").

What should you do if you encounter a negative or potentially aggressive situation with someone? Consider the following example: your partner tells you that they do not want to have a discussion, or keeps putting off the day/ time to talk.

The acronym FAST is made up of four skills you can use to validate your own thoughts, feelings, or desires and maintain self-respect.

- *(Be) Fair:* As much as the situation or response may hurt or upset you, be fair to yourself by validating your own thoughts and feelings, and those of the other person (e.g., "I hear what you are saying/I know this is going to be hard for both of us; however, I want us to improve our relationship").
- *(No) Apologies:* While it is important to apologize in certain circumstances, you do not need to continuously apologize. For example, you do not need to apologize to your partner for wanting to have a conversation about your relationship. Avoid looking down at the floor or looking embarrassed. Maintain eye contact and an erect posture.
- *Stick to values:* Be true to your thoughts and feelings. You have had a relationship with your partner for X amount of time, and you love them. You do not have to walk away with your head down. Explain the aforementioned point.
- *(Be) Truthful:* Do not lie/manipulate (e.g., "Well, I guess you must be seeing someone else, since I'm clearly not important to you"), exaggerate or be dramatic (e.g., "If you don't talk to me/if we don't improve our relationship, I'm going to kill myself"; "Fine! I'll just go find someone else who will appreciate me"), minimize (e.g., "I guess it's fine. We don't really need to talk") or act helpless (e.g., "I cannot live without you").

Group Activity: Draw a "pros and cons" list on the whiteboard and ask clients to list the pros and cons of not using DEAR MAN skills. Ask them to look at the lists and share whether they think these skills could be useful for them to use. Why or why not?

Skills Trainer: GIVE FAST Skills

Relationships can be challenging if you tend to respond in a passive, aggressive, or passive-aggressive manner. Let's look at the skills below and use the following example:

> *You typically come home from work around 5:00 pm. One night, you decide to hang out with your friends for an hour after work without letting your partner/spouse know. When you get home, your partner is upset because you a) are late coming home, and b) did not contact them to let them know where you were.*

Review the handout, GIVE FAST Skills, with participants and ask if they have questions.

> *Be prepared that you may not get the answer you want. For example, it is possible that your partner is pulling away because they want to break up. At this point, you will have to accept their position no matter how painful it is. Remember that radical acceptance is not about pushing your feelings away, but rather accepting them as they are in the moment, and eventually letting them go.*

Roleplay: Ask clients to find a partner. Partner A will share a personal scenario where they did not use their GIVE FAST skills but could have. Both partners will reenact the scenario, only this time Partner A will use their GIVE FAST skills. After completing this, partners will switch places and Partner B will then share a personal scenario to reenact.

Handout 11.1: DEAR MAN

- **Describe the current interaction:** When we feel frustrated by an interaction, we tend to react to others using our emotion mind. In a frustrating interaction, explain why you are feeling the way you do using only facts (e.g., "I've noticed that we haven't been as close as we used to be").
- **Express thoughts or feelings about the interaction:** For example, "I feel sad/badly that we haven't been communicating well."
- **Assert wishes in the situation:** For example, "I would really like to improve our relationship, and I think sitting down and calmly talking about our issues would be helpful").
- **Reinforce:** "Reinforcement" refers to rewarding the other person for doing what you want. You may need to address negative consequences here, too (e.g., "I want to make things good again between us." If necessary, "Because I love you and want us both to be happy"). Reinforcement should also include verbal and/or non-verbal communication after you get what you want (e.g., smile, thank the person, give them a hug if they consent to it. Make sure they are aware that they have done something helpful, and that you are appreciative).
- **Mindful of needs:** Stay mindful of your boundaries, and those of others. Avoid distractions around you, or from the other person. Stick to the topic!
- **Appear confident:** You do not have to feel confident, but it is important to present yourself as such. For example, stand up straight, make good eye contact, and speak clearly and directly.
- **Negotiate:** Negotiation is not manipulation; it is a give-and-take solution to the problem (e.g., your partner does not have time to talk right now. Let them know that you would like to talk when they have time. Ask them if you can both agree on a good time to have the conversation). Asking for a concrete day/time means that you are serious about having a conversation, yet also flexible.

Handout 11.2: GIVE FAST Skills

- **(Be) <u>G</u>entle:** Being gentle during interactions is a means of being respectful. In other words, it means that you do not judge (e.g., "My partner is so needy that they can't let me go out for an hour with my friends), threaten (e.g., "You're just making me want leave and go back to hang out with them"), attack (e.g., "Why can't you ever cut me break? All you do is nag me!"), or completely dismiss what the other person is saying (e.g., walking away).
- **(Act) <u>I</u>nterested:** This does not necessarily mean that you are interested in what the other person is saying, but rather that you act as though you are. When someone acts interested, they:
  - Actively listen to the other person's point of view.
  - Make eye contact with the other person (e.g., avoid looking down, around you, or at your phone).
  - Do not interrupt the other person; wait until they are done talking to respond.
- **<u>V</u>alidate:** Validation is the recognition of another person's thoughts and feelings.
  - Consider how you might feel if you were in the other person's shoes.
  - Avoid taking a defensive stance.
  - Repeat what you heard the other person say (e.g., "I understand why you are upset with me. I should have called you to let you know I was going out with my friends").
- **(Use an) <u>E</u>asy manner:** Put the other person at ease rather than being defensive, or having an attitude. You may want to touch your partner's hand and move closer with them to let them know you care about their feelings. You could also say something humorous to ease the tension (e.g., "This aging thing is no joke. I can't even remember what I had for breakfast this morning. I've got to do better").
- **(Be) <u>F</u>air:** As much as the situation or response may hurt or upset you, be fair to yourself by validating your own thoughts and feelings, and those of the other person (e.g., "I hear what you are saying/I know this is going to be hard for both of us; however, I want us to improve our relationship").
- **(No) <u>A</u>pologies:** While it is important to apologize in certain circumstances, you do not need to continuously apologize. For example, you do not need to apologize to your partner for wanting to have a

conversation about your relationship. Avoid looking down at the floor or looking embarrassed. Maintain eye contact and an erect posture.

- **<u>S</u>tick to values:** Be true to your thoughts and feelings. You have had a relationship with your partner for X amount of time, and you love them. You do not have to walk away with your head down. Explain the aforementioned point.

  - **(Be) <u>T</u>ruthful:** Do not lie/manipulate (e.g., "Well, I guess you must be seeing someone else, since I'm clearly not important to you"), exaggerate or be dramatic (e.g., "If you don't talk to me/if we don't improve our relationship, I'm going to kill myself"; "Fine! I'll just go find someone else who will appreciate me"), minimize (e.g., "I guess it's fine. We don't really need to talk") or act helpless (e.g., "I cannot live without you").

Note

1 Alleyene (2009).

References

Alleyene R. (2009). Talking to plants makes them grow, especially if you are a woman, according to an experiment by the Royal Horticultural Society. *The Telegraph.* https://www.telegraph.co.uk/news/earth/earthnews/5602419/Womens-voices-make-plants-grow-faster-finds-Royal-Horticultural-Society.html

Interpersonal Effectiveness Skills in Relationships and Relationship Barriers

12

Skills Trainer:
Research shows that there are four major factors that can erode and eventually ruin a relationship.[1] A psychologist couple, John and Julie Gottman, studied people and their romantic relationships for years, and refer to these factors—criticism, contempt, defensiveness, and stonewalling—as "The Four Horsemen."

Group Activity: Review Handout 12.1: The Four Horsemen in depth and ask participants to provide an example from their lives.

Criticism

Criticism is different from expressing your thoughts and feelings in a healthy, non-threatening way (DEAR MAN, GIVE FAST), in that it is an attack on your partner's very being. Consider the following example: you want to have more sexual intimacy with your partner, but they are content having sex once or twice a month. You interpret this as your partner not being attracted to you, and that makes you feel hurt and upset. You say to your partner, "We used to have sex all the time; now you never want it. That is not what a good partner does." In essence, you are using an emotional response to blame your partner and make them feel badly about themselves. This is problematic in a relationship because the other person feels personally attacked. Criticizing your partner—rather than using your interpersonal effectiveness skills—may lead

DOI: 10.4324/9781003451099-16

to them feeling contempt for you, becoming defensive, or simply walking away and ignoring you.

Defensiveness

Responding to another person in a defensive manner typically leads to an argument or fight. People usually become defensive when they are criticized— or perceive they have been criticized, without confirming the other person's intentions. Consider the criticism of your partner above ("We used to have sex all the time; now you never want it. That is not what a good partner does"). Your partner is hurt by your criticism, and responds, "You know that I work long hours, and I have to take care of the kids; how dare you demand anything else from me." As most people respond to criticism or perceived criticism defensively, the problem is that each partner now feels attacked, so the vicious circle continues.

Contempt

Showing contempt for someone is different from criticizing them. While criticism is an attack on your partner, contempt is when someone treats their partner as worthless, or "less-than ..." Treating someone with contempt can be done verbally (e.g., mocking others; calling them names); non-verbally (e.g., eyerolling; making sounds that indicate you do not respect what they are saying); or through behavior (e.g., undermining someone's work or role; being deceptive). Let's continue to use the previous example. You ask your partner to have sex with you. Your partner declines because they are tired. You roll your eyes and say something like, "Of course you are. You're always too tired for everything"; "You're so lazy and dumb"; or "Fine—I'll just go to the bar and meet a woman who actually knows how to be a woman." Behaving with contempt is disrespectful because it creates a power dynamic between you and your partner, and leads them to feelings of worthlessness and self-doubt.

Stonewalling

Stonewalling typically happens when someone has experienced ongoing criticism and / or contempt. "Stonewalling" refers to shutting down emotionally, walking away from someone, tuning them out, or pretending to be busy instead of discussing the issue. For example, you frequently criticize your partner or treat them with contempt when you do not get what you want. Your partner eventually gets fed up with your demeaning comments and tunes you out or walks away when they sense you getting angry. Once a relationship reaches this point, it is difficult to repair the harm because it has already created a significant rift between you.

Skills Trainer:

You may have heard other people talk about or encourage you to make a "list" of what you are looking for in a relationship. However, a few problems arise when making these lists. First, people tend to be vague. For example, they might say that they are looking for someone with whom they have "good communication"; or a relationship that is "loving" and "giving." These terms are quite vague and do not address the specific interactions and behaviors you need for a healthy and happy relationship. Second, when people make these lists, they tend to add standards or preferences they are looking for, such as "blonde hair," "thin," or "makes more than $100,000 a year." While you may be attracted to thin people with blonde hair, does that mean you can't be open to someone who has a curvy or athletic build, has brown hair, but also possesses qualities you deem important in a relationship?

Instead of completing a list of what you want, making a list of your non-negotiables—what you cannot tolerate in a person or relationship—is more effective in terms of finding a partner that has the qualities you want for a happy relationship. "Non-negotiables" are what you are absolutely unwilling to accept in a relationship. For example, instead of looking for a partner who earns a specific salary, one of your non-negotiables may be that your partner is financially stable—in other words, they pay their bills on time and are responsible with their money. Instead of saying that you want "good communication," describe what you would like that to look like. In this instance, your non-negotiable might be "no name calling," "no yelling and screaming when we disagree," or "no 'Four Horsemen' behaviors."

Practice Exercise: Ask participants to write down their non-negotiables with respect to relationships. After they have finished, write their responses on the whiteboard. You will likely receive some responses that do not sound like "non-negotiables." If this arises, probe the client for further clarification, and gently encourage them to consider how their response might translate into a non-negotiable one.

Skills Trainer:

Making friends or meeting a potential partner is important, and it is up to you to initiate the process. People tend to enjoy spending time with those who have similar interests. When meeting people, what are some behaviors you may want to avoid?

Examples:

- *Oversharing personal information.*
- *Asking too many personal questions.*
- *Being overly negative.*
- *Lying about who you are and what your interests are, so you seem more compatible.*
- *Invading the other's personal space.*
- *Making sexual comments about the person or others.*

Disclosure

Determining the right time to disclose your offense is hard, and even the thought of disclosing can cause a lot of anxiety. It is not recommended that you disclose your offense the first time you meet someone. Instead, spend time getting to know them platonically. If you are spending time with someone with whom you are interested in having a relationship, go on a few dates first. While there is no specific amount of time to wait, it is extremely important that you disclose your offense to a potential partner prior to having sex with them. It is important for them to know so they can make an informed decision about how they want to proceed in the relationship. In addition, if the person has custody of their children, and you have probation conditions that prohibit you from being around minors, you may want to reconsider having a relationship with them. If you have any questions about disclosure, be sure to talk to your individual therapist or discuss them in group.

Skills Trainer: Review Handout 12.2: Meeting People, Making Friends, and Disclosure with clients. Next, ask group members to fill out Handout 12.3: Developing My Boundaries and Respecting Others. This may take 20–30 minutes. Be sure to walk around the room to answer clients' questions and provide them with feedback. After completing the exercise, ask each client to read their responses to one or two of the scenarios in the handout. Encourage the group to provide each other with feedback.

In the coming week, clients will apply the concepts acquired in Chapter 11 as they complete Handouts 12.4: Interpersonal Effectiveness Skills, Past Offending, and My Relationships and 12.5: My Intimacy Ladders.

Handout 12.1: The Four Horsemen

- **Criticism**

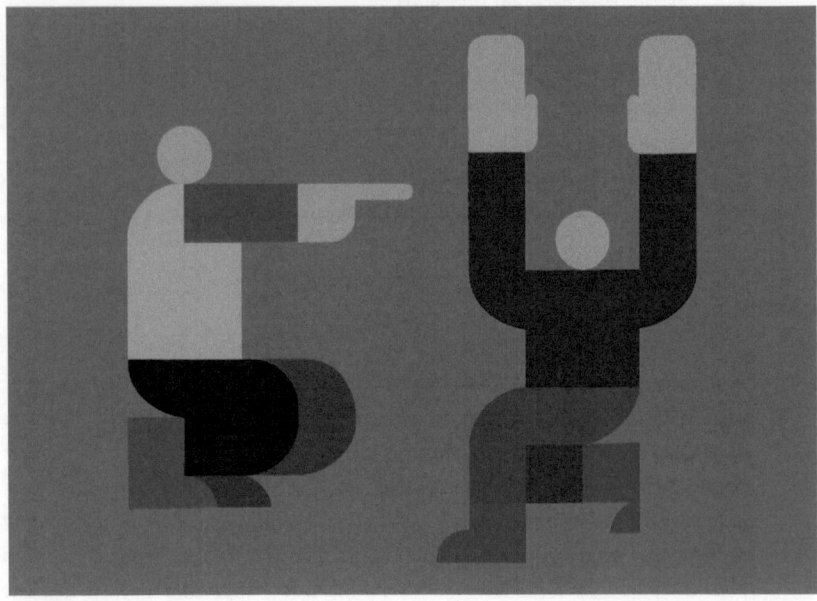

Image 12.1 Person pointing a finger at another person whose hands are raised

"The blame game:"
Credit: Kareena S. https://paintyourblues.com/guidelines/

- **Defensiveness**

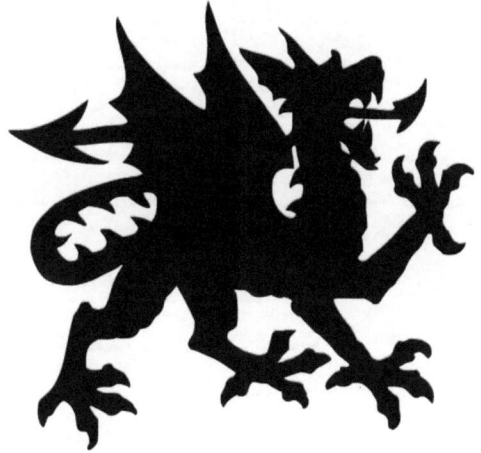

Image 12.2 Dragon

- **Contempt**

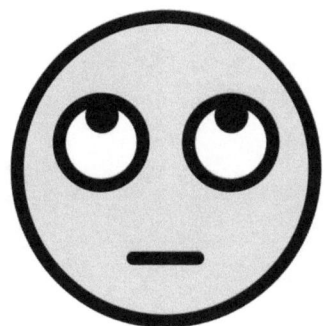

Image 12.3 Rolling Eyes

- **Stonewalling**

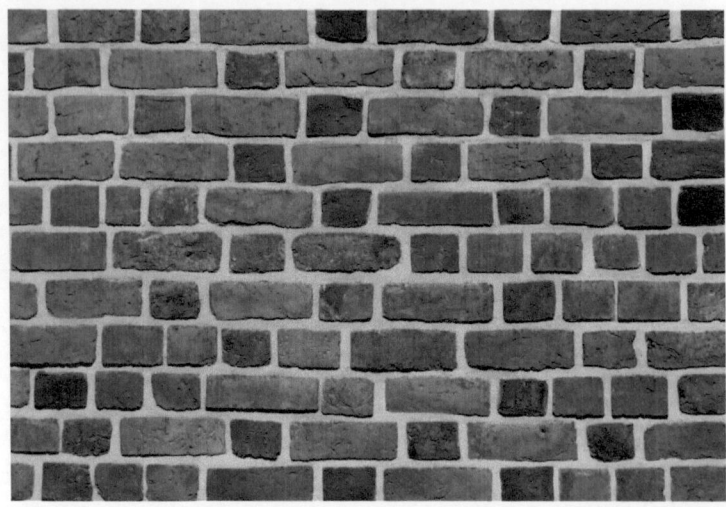

Image 12.4 Brick wall

Handout 12.2: Meeting People, Making Friends, and Disclosure

Ideas to Meet Friends/A Potential Partner

It is important to interact with others who share similar interests as you (e.g., hiking, reading, writing, gardening). Meetup.com is a good place to start.

If you do not have access to the Internet, contact your local library or university to find out if they host adult-friendly events or groups. You can also ask your individual therapist to look up groups for you, or to provide you with a phone number or a meetup location.

- Go to a restaurant or cafe by yourself for food or coffee. If the opportunity presents itself, chat with someone sitting near you. Keep the conversation light and pay attention to their body language. They may not want to talk to you but are uncomfortable saying "no." Sometimes restaurants and cafes post flyers about upcoming events, or adult group get-togethers.
- Attend a religious institution. Ask about adult group events and activities.
- Ask a friend or adult family member if you can spend time with them when they hang out with people you do not know.
- Other ideas:

_____

_____

_____

_____

_____

_____

_____

Where *Not* to Meet Potential Partners

- **Jail/prison:** You meet these people under adverse circumstances. You both have engaged in law-breaking behavior. Forming and maintaining long-term relationships with negative peers is a risk factor for reoffending.
- **Halfway house:** Similar to the above. Two people with criminal histories, histories of engaging in high-risk behavior, or other challenges will typically influence one another.
- **Self-help groups (e.g., Alcoholics Anonymous, Narcotics Anonymous, Sex Addicts Anonymous):** These people are struggling with the same issues as you, or may be struggling even more. When one partner relapses, it is common for the other to relapse too.
- Other ideas:

_____

_____

_____

_____

_____

_____

Handout 12.3: Developing My Boundaries and Respecting Others

- **Me (to my parole officer):** *"Officer, I would really like to get a computer to keep a journal and send emails. Would this be possible?"*
- **Parole officer:** *"No. You are not allowed to have internet access; nor can you be in possession of a computer, even if it doesn't have internet access."*

My response: _____

- **My partner:** *"I am fed up that we can't do the things I want to do because you committed this offense and now have all of the conditions to follow for probation."*

My response: _____

- **My neighbor:** *"You're a sex offender! If you so much as say 'hi' to my children, I will call the police."*

My response: _____

- **My friend:** *"I know you're supposed to be home when you're not at work, but I really need a ride to see my mom. Please help me out just this one time."*

My response: _____

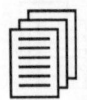

Handout 12.4: Interpersonal Effectiveness Skills, Past Offending, and My Relationships

Part 1: Consider the various interpersonal effectiveness skills listed in Handout 9.1: Interpersonal Skills Rating Scale. Explain how failing to use these skills led to you committing your offense(s). List each sexual offense you have committed. If there are more than three offenses, list the others on the back of the page. If your offense involved possession and/or distribution of child sexual exploitation material, list three times you engaged in this behavior and respond to the questions below.

  Part II: Once you have completed this part, list at least one negative relationship or interaction you have had with (a) a romantic partner or romantic interest, (b) the legal system, and (c) family/friends. Then consider a time in the relationship when you demonstrated a lack of interpersonal effectiveness skills and describe that situation. Once you have done this, write what skills you will use and how you will use them to address this situation if it arises again. Only write down skills that you can commit to using.

Part I: Offenses

Offense #1

How my actions demonstrated a lack of interpersonal effectiveness skills:

_____

_____

_____

_____

_____

How I will use my interpersonal effectiveness skills to avoid being in this situation again:

_____

_____

_____

_____

_____

Offense #2

How my actions demonstrated a lack of interpersonal effectiveness skills:

_____

_____

_____

_____

_____

How I will use my interpersonal effectiveness skills to avoid being in this situation again:

_____

_____

_____

_____

_____

Offense #3

How my actions demonstrated a lack of interpersonal effectiveness skills:

_____

_____

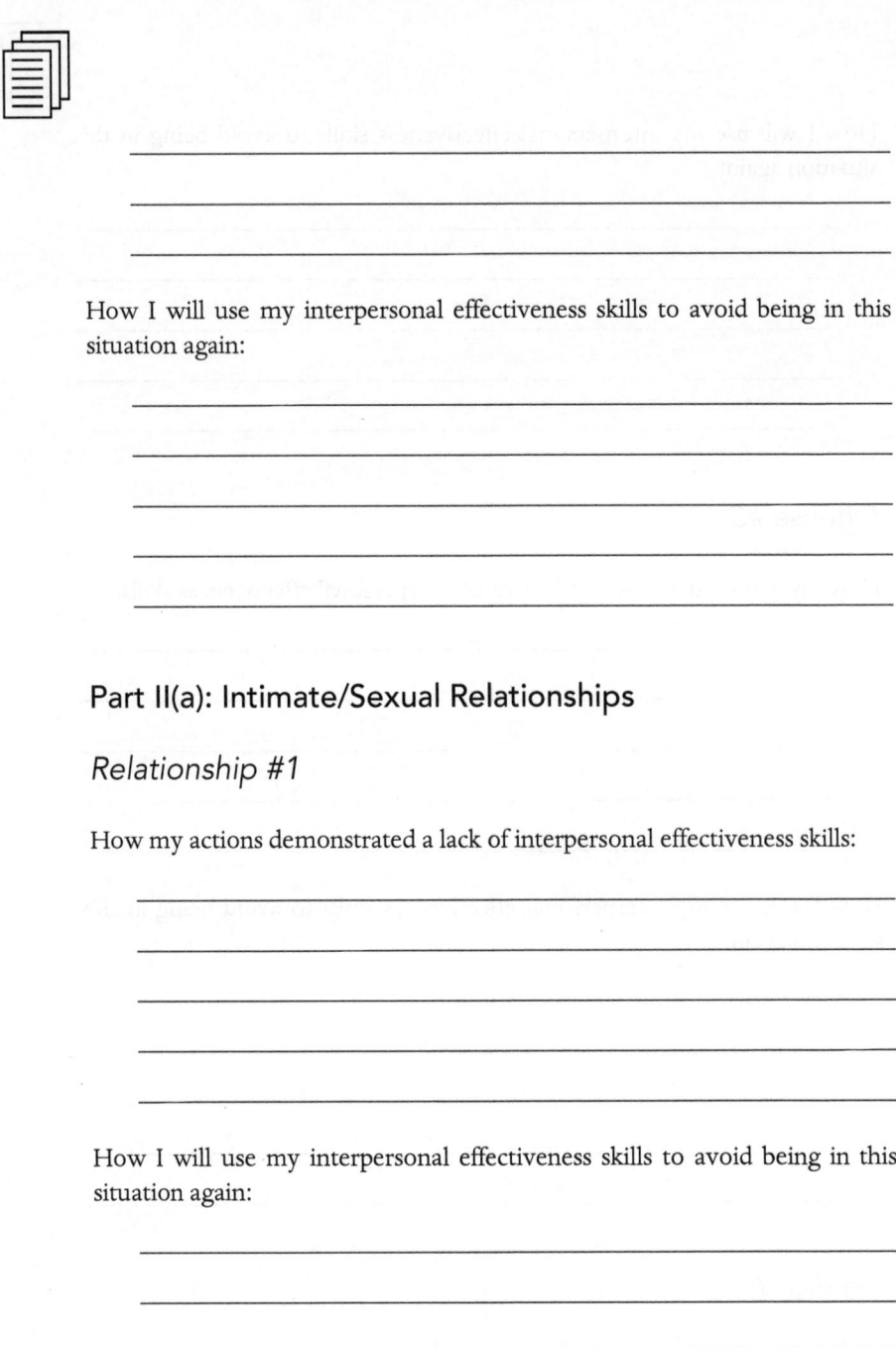

_____

_____

_____

How I will use my interpersonal effectiveness skills to avoid being in this situation again:

_____

_____

_____

_____

Part II(a): Intimate/Sexual Relationships

Relationship #1

How my actions demonstrated a lack of interpersonal effectiveness skills:

_____

_____

_____

_____

How I will use my interpersonal effectiveness skills to avoid being in this situation again:

_____

_____

_____

_____

Relationship #2

How my actions demonstrated a lack of interpersonal effectiveness skills:

_____

_____

_____

_____

_____

How I will use my interpersonal effectiveness skills to avoid being in this situation again:

_____

_____

_____

_____

_____

Relationship #3

How my actions demonstrated a lack of interpersonal effectiveness skills:

_____

_____

_____

_____

_____

How I will use my interpersonal effectiveness skills to avoid being in this situation again:

_____

_____

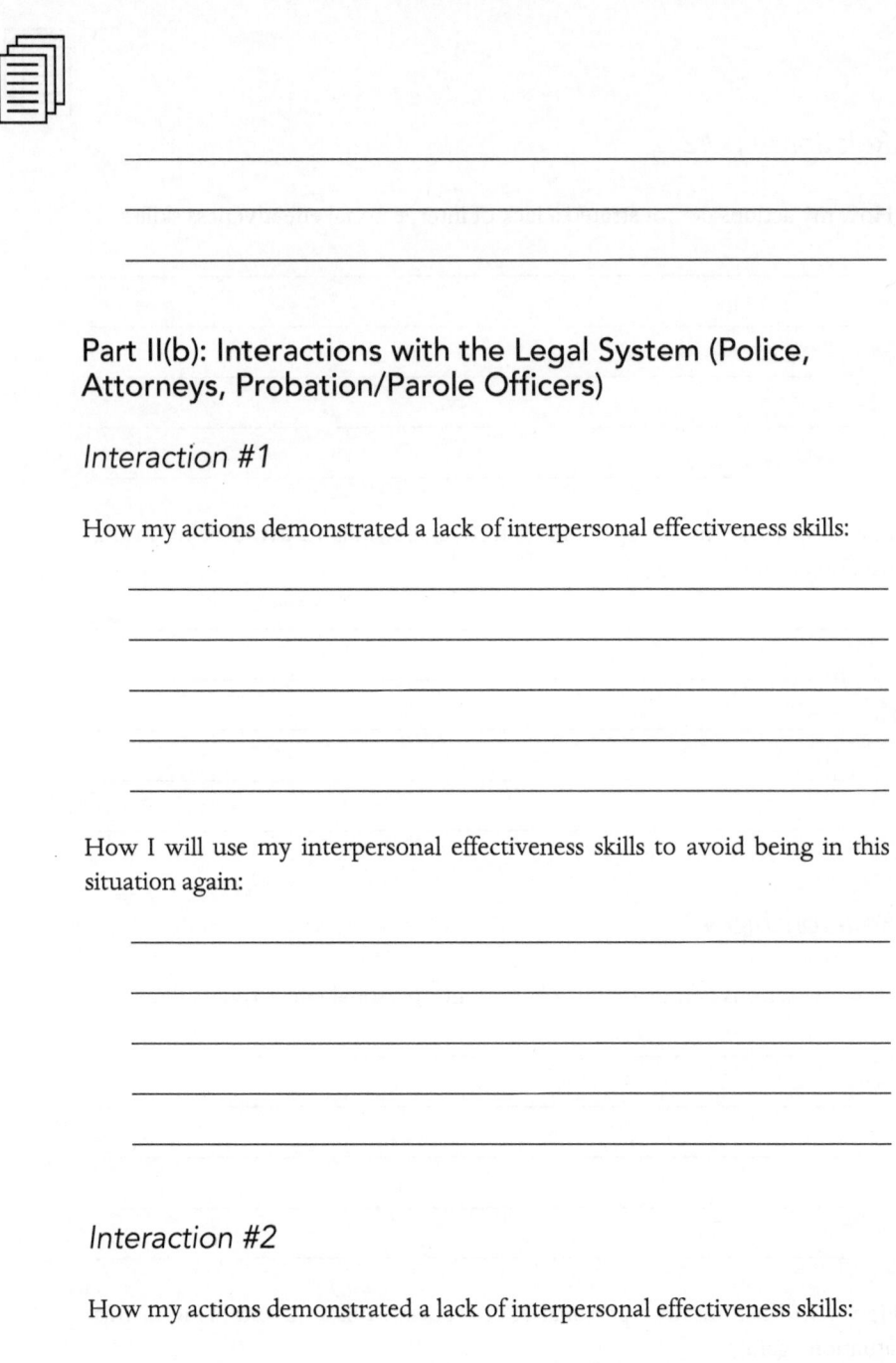

_____

_____

_____

Part II(b): Interactions with the Legal System (Police, Attorneys, Probation/Parole Officers)

Interaction #1

How my actions demonstrated a lack of interpersonal effectiveness skills:

_____

_____

_____

_____

_____

How I will use my interpersonal effectiveness skills to avoid being in this situation again:

_____

_____

_____

_____

_____

Interaction #2

How my actions demonstrated a lack of interpersonal effectiveness skills:

_____

_____

_____

_____

_____

How I will use my interpersonal effectiveness skills to avoid being in this situation again:

_____

_____

_____

_____

_____

Interaction #3

How my actions demonstrated a lack of interpersonal effectiveness skills:

_____

_____

_____

_____

_____

How I will use my interpersonal effectiveness skills to avoid being in this situation again:

_____

_____

_____

_____

_____

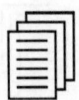

Part II(c): Interpersonal Relationship Effectiveness and Interactions with Friends and Family

Relationship #1

How my actions demonstrated a lack of interpersonal effectiveness skills:

_____

_____

_____

_____

How I will use my interpersonal effectiveness skills to avoid being in this situation again:

_____

_____

_____

_____

_____

Relationship #2

How my actions demonstrated a lack of interpersonal effectiveness skills:

_____

_____

_____

_____

_____

How I will use my interpersonal effectiveness skills to avoid being in this situation again:

_____

_____

_____

_____

_____

Relationship #3

How my actions demonstrated a lack of interpersonal effectiveness skills:

_____

_____

_____

_____

_____

How I will use my interpersonal effectiveness skills to avoid being in this situation again:

_____

_____

_____

_____

_____

Handout 12.5: My Intimacy Ladders

"Intimacy" is defined as emotional closeness. In other words, it is not just sexual in nature. Intimacy can increase or decrease depending on the types of relationships you have with various people in your lives. Think about your relationships with others—past or present. These relationships can include partners, children, family, friends, associates, coworkers... Not everyone has high levels of intimacy with their partners, or family. On the other hand, some people misinterpret the behavior of strangers or acquaintances as intimacy. Draw an arrow from each individual listed under the "People" section to one of the rungs on the ladder to indicate how much intimacy/emotional closeness you feel with them. Next, you will answer questions about barriers to these relationships. Finally, you will complete two more intimacy ladders—one that addresses how you think the individuals listed below view their intimacy with you, and the other addressing the levels of intimacy you would like to have.

High Intimacy

HIGH INTIMACY

LOW INTIMACY

People:

Mother/Father

Siblings

Children

Friends?

Co-workers

Neighbors

Extended family members

Anyone else?

Image 12.5 Ladder

Low Intimacy

List some of the barriers to your relationships with the following people (e.g., do you struggle to share your thoughts and feelings?)

1. _____

2. _____

3. _____

4. _____

5. _____

6. _____

7. _____

8. _____

9. _____

10. _____

Now, consider the same list of people and place each person on the rung that indicates how you think *they* view their level of intimacy with you:

HIGH INTIMACY

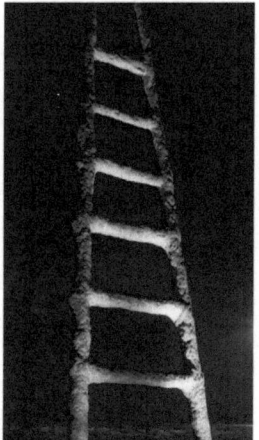

LOW INTIMACY

People:

Mother/Father

Siblings

Children

Friends?

Co-workers

Neighbors

Extended family members

Anyone else?

Copyright material from Abigail Kolb, *Dialectical Behavior Therapy for Sex Offenders: A Treatment Guide*, 2024, Routledge

Is there a discrepancy in terms of your perceived level of intimacy and others' perceived levels? List the reasons why this might be:

1. _____
2. _____
3. _____
4. _____
5. _____
6. _____
7. _____
8. _____
9. _____
10. _____

Finally, use the same list to place each person on the rung that indicates where you *would like them to be* in your life:

HIGH INTIMACY

People:

Mother/Father

Siblings

Children

Friends?

Co-workers

Neighbors

Extended family members

Anyone else?

LOW INTIMACY

Image 12.5 Ladder

Credit: Hans22, CC BY-SA 3.0 NL https://creativecommons.org/licenses/by-sa/3.0/nl/deed.en

What do you need to do to make your relationships match what you would like to have?

1. _____

2. _____

3. _____

4. _____

5. _____

6. _____

7. _____

8. _____

9. _____

10. _____

Note

1 Gottman (1993).

Reference

Gottman J. M. (1993). The roles of conflict engagement, escalation, and avoidance in marital interaction: A longitudinal view of five types of couples. *Journal of Consulting and Clinical Psychology, 61*(1), 6–15. https://doi.org/10.1037//0022-006X.61.1.6

Emotion Regulation Skills

Part IV

Empathy[1]   **13**

Group Activity: When learning to write an essay in school, we start by writing the introduction. This paragraph provides the basic structure for the rest of the paper; it is a framework. At the end of the introductory paragraph, you must have a statement that focuses the paper, so the reader knows what the focus of the paper will be. Tell clients to take out a piece of paper and a pen.

Now, write an introductory paragraph about your life right now. Who are you? The thesis statement, or the end of your paragraph, should end with three or four values you hold, and what you need to do to live by these values.

If clients struggle with writing, you can have them draw instead.

Skills Trainer: *Ask clients to share their paragraph.*

In order to live by your values and not reoffend, it is important to understand the experiences of others in various contexts, or "put yourself in another person's shoes," regardless of how you think they should respond.[2] This is referred to as "empathy." Failing to empathize with others, and focusing only on one's own needs, will lead to further barriers in relationships. When this happens, it can lead to rejection, loneliness, sexualization of children, anger toward women, self-pity, and depression—factors that led to your offense in the first place. As you know, sexual offenses are violations of others' boundaries and overall wellbeing. While you may not lack empathy in general, when you committed your offense(s), you demonstrated a lack of empathy for your victim(s), their loved ones, your loved ones, and the community at large. In order to empathize

DOI: 10.4324/9781003451099-18

with others, you first have to understand your thinking errors before, during, and after the offense, and accept responsibility for your actions.

Victims of sexual abuse experience short and long-term consequences as a result of the abuse they experienced. Some of these include:

- *Revictimization: Research shows that some individuals who have been victimized may experience changes in their non-verbal communication, such as walking with their head down; and changes in daily routines and activities[3] that may place them at greater harm—all of which has been shown to help offenders identify potential victims.[4]*
- *Problems with mental health, including depression, anxiety, substance abuse, trauma responses, and self-harm and suicide.[5]*
- *Self-imposed isolation/problems making and maintaining relationships with others.[6]*
- *Higher rates of teen pregnancy and promiscuity.[7]*
- *Fear of sexual intimacy.[8]*
- *Victimization of others.[9]*

Roleplay—Humanizing the Victim(s): For this activity, ask participants to split into groups of two. Person A will assume the role of the victim and tell Person B (who will assume the role of offender) how the offense affected them during and after the offending period. Explain that Person A should attempt to identify the victim's thoughts, emotions, physical feelings, and actions (e.g., had to talk to the police; go to court; go to the doctor/hospital for a rape kit; suffered anal or vaginal tearing or other injuries sustained during the offense; had to take medication to prevent sexually transmitted infections; had to have therapy, etc.). Next, Person A and Person B will switch places, so Person B has the opportunity to assume the role of the victim(s). Once they have completed the exercise, ask clients to rejoin the group and share their thoughts and emotions about the activity. Engage in discussion about the activity.

Notes:

- If the client used child sexual exploitation material, they should consider two or three different victims in the images they viewed to account for context.
- If the client victimized the same person more than once, they should identify how the victim may have felt throughout the offending period.
- If the client has multiple victims, they should play the role of each victim, as the context may have been different.

Handout 13.1: Empathy

For your homework, you will complete a behavior chain analysis (BCA) about your offense. However, in this BCA, the consequences will reflect the consequences to the victims.

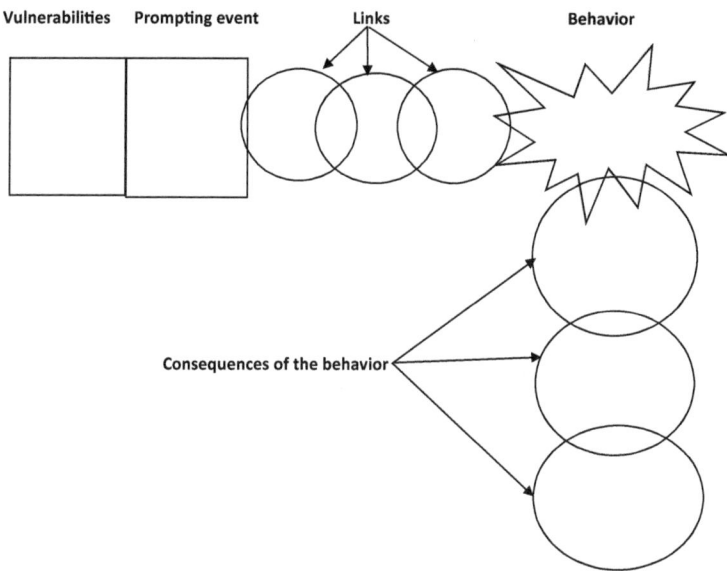

First, list the events that triggered your offending (i.e., the precursors. What was going on in your life at the time?)

_____

_____

_____

_____

Next, list your beliefs about what was going on in your life. What were your beliefs about yourself, those around you, your relationships, your victim(s), and your action(s)?

_____

_____

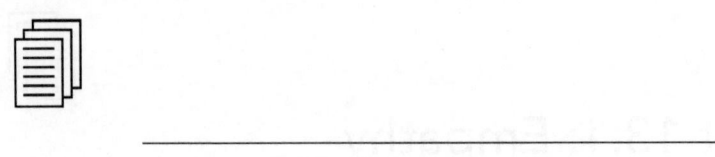

_____

_____

List the long-term and short-term consequences of your offending behavior:
How do you think your actions affected the person you abused?

_____

_____

_____

_____

_____

_____

How do you think your actions affected your victim's family (consider
physical, emotional/psychological, social, educational, and financial effects)?

_____

_____

_____

_____

_____

_____

How do you think your actions affected your family?

_____

_____

_____

_____

_____

_____

_____

_____

How do you think your actions affected society?

_____

_____

_____

_____

_____

_____

_____

List behaviors you must avoid, and behaviors you must do in order to avoid negative consequences in the future:

Behaviors	Avoid	Do

Notes

1 Note: Be mindful of antisocial/psychopathic clients who are unable to feel empathy for their victims. Instead, I engage these clients in strictly cognitive-behavioral methods such as asking them to identify the short and long-term consequences of their behaviors on their lives, and actions they must take or avoid in order to avoid unwanted consequences in the future (see Handout 13.1: Empathy).
2 Ward & Durrant (2013).
3 Lauritsen & Quinet (1995); Wittebrood & Nieuwbeerta (2000).
4 Stuart, Smodis, & Forth (2022).
5 Trickett, Noll, & Putnam (2011).
6 Trickett, Noll, & Putnam (2011).
7 Widom, & Kuhns (1996).
8 Trickett, Noll, & Putnam (2011).
9 Hanson & Slater (1988).

References

Galietta M. M., & Rosenfeld B. (2012). Adapting dialectical behavior therapy (DBT) for the treatment of psychopathy. *International Journal of Forensic Mental Health, 11,* 325–335.

Guo P., Wang M., Cheng C., & Chen H. (2022). Psychopathic dispositions and emotion dysregulation: A dual-disposition model perspective. *Journal of Clinical Psychology, 78*(6), 1170–1183. https://doi.org/10.1002/jclp.23274

Hanson R. K., & Slater S. (1988). Sexual victimization in the history of sexual abusers: A review. *Annals of Sex Research, 1*(4), 485–499. https://doi.org/10.1007/BF00854712

Hare R. D. (2003). *The Hare Psychopathy Checklist—Revised* (2nd ed.). Toronto: Multi-Health Systems.

Hare R. D. (1991). *Manual for the Revised Psychopathy Checklist* (1st ed.). Toronto: Multi-Health Systems.

Hare R. D., & Neumann C. S. (2008). Psychopathy as a clinical and empirical construct. *Annual Review of Clinical Psychology, 4*, 217–246. https://doi.org/10.1146/annurev.clinpsy.3.022806.091452

Lauritsen J. L., & Quinet K. F. (1995). Repeat victimization among adolescents and young adults. *Journal of Quantitative Criminology, 11*(2), 143–166. https://doi.org/10.1007/BF02221121

Linehan M. M (1993). *Cognitive-Behavioral Treatment of Borderline Personality Disorder.* New York: Guilford Publications.

Stuart J., Smodis A., & Forth A. (2022). Perceived personality traits and presumptions of vulnerability to victimization in women. *Journal of Criminal Psychology, 12*(6). http://doi.org/10.1108/JCP-04-2021-0011

Trickett P. K., Noll J. G., & Putnam F. W. (2011). The impact of sexual abuse on female development: Lessons from a multigenerational, longitudinal research study. *Development and Psychopathology, 23*(2), 453–476. https://doi.org/10.1017/S0954579411000174

Ward T., & Durrant R. (2013). Altruism, empathy, and sex offender treatment. *International Journal of Behavioral Consultation and Therapy, 8*(3–4), 66–71. https://doi.org/10.1037/h0100986

Widom C. S., & Kuhns J. B. (1996). Childhood victimization and subsequent risk for promiscuity, prostitution, and teenage pregnancy: A prospective study. *American Journal of Public Health, 86*(11), 1607–1612. https://doi.org/10.2105/ajph.86.11.1607

Wittebrood K., & Nieuwbeerta P. (2000). Criminal victimization during one's life course: The effects of previous victimization and patterns of routine activities. *Journal of Research in Crime and Delinquency, 37*(1), 91–122. https://doi.org/10.1177/0022427800037001004

Acknowledging, Identifying, and Regulating Emotions

14

Skills Trainer:

The purpose of emotion regulation is not to avoid having feelings, but to identify and describe your emotions, reduce your suffering when you experience a negative emotion, and decrease the frequency of unwanted emotions.

Note: Galietta and Rosenfield (2012) have made important modifications to dialectical behavioral therapy in their work with individuals with psychopathic personality traits; and while their results are not currently generalizable, they found that teaching these individuals emotion regulation skills did yield positive outcomes.[1]

Group Discussion: Draw a table like the one below on the whiteboard and then follow these five steps:

- Ask participants to share what they think they could gain from emotion regulation skills and list responses in the first column.
- Ask participants about any negative outcomes that could stem from using emotion regulation skills and list responses in the second column.
- Ask participants what they have gained from instances when they did not control their emotions and list responses in the third column.
- Ask participants what they have gained by regulating their emotions and list responses in the fourth column.
- Finally, ask each participant which emotions they want to learn to regulate, and how they think emotion regulation skills could benefit them.

DOI: 10.4324/9781003451099-19

Benefits of using emotion regulation skills	Consequences/ negative outcomes from using emotion regulation skills	What I have gained by *not* controlling my emotions	What I have gained by regulating my emotions

Skills Trainer:

There are many myths about emotions and men may feel particularly vulnerable as a result. Take out Handout 14.1: Myths I Have about Emotions, and check the boxes that apply to your beliefs about emotions. Then, write a challenge statement you can tell yourself so you do not fall into the "emotional thinking errors trap". It is important to learn emotion regulation skills because emotions play a role in our everyday lives, and in our relationships. Emotions serve various functions, including helping us communicate how we feel to ourselves and others. Showing emotions does not make you weak; it can actually help improve your interpersonal relationships. However, sometimes people get stuck in emotion mind and express extreme emotions; or emotions can be harmful and create problems in their lives. Unhealthy or illegal behaviors that stem from negative emotions can be reinforced, and become hard to change as a result. This means that your thoughts, emotions, and behaviors stemming from the event felt good, at least initially. We tend to repeat behaviors that make us feel good; this is referred to as "reinforcement." Consider the following examples:

- *John feels bored so he masturbates to pornography. John has an orgasm and feels better. John is now more likely to use pornography to make himself feel better when he has a negative emotion.*

- Carlos feels lonely and depressed, so he goes online to find a person to "hook up" with. He goes to the person's home, has sex with them, and immediately feels better. However, having sex without intimacy, in addition to a continued lack of a permanent partner, leads him back to his feelings of loneliness and depression. Having sex without intimacy makes him feel better in the moment, but it ultimately contributes to the very emotions he is trying to escape.
- Michael feels good when he goes to the park, pulls down his pants, and masturbates publicly. He knows his behavior is illegal and wrong, but whenever he feels anxious or sad, he engages in this behavior to make himself feel better. Once he has finished masturbating and goes home, Michael feels disgusted by his actions and tells himself that he is a loser, so he drinks vodka until he falls asleep.

In the third scenario, Michael is using a sexual behavior to cope with his negative emotions. The behavior makes him feel good in the moment, but it also leads to him feeling shame after. Why does Michael continue to do this behavior when it makes him feel worse than he did before doing it?

This happens when an individual's behavior has been reinforced. In this case, Michael has learned, through reinforcement (the orgasm and the belief that someone who sees his penis might be turned on), that his behavior makes him feel good. Not only does the orgasm feel good, but Michael believes it is possible that a woman walking past him will find him attractive and want to date him, or at least have sex with him. These reinforcements may be so strong that they outweigh the negative consequences in the end. In other words, this initial reaction to a negative feeling served a function for Michael because it made him feel better in the moment. However, Michael does not like the feelings he experiences after engaging in the behavior. He is also fearful that he might get arrested.

Many people act on their emotions rather than thinking things through rationally. Remember that **feelings are not facts**! This means that your emotions are not necessarily factual, but rather the way you have perceived an event. Think back to your offense staircase and recall how situations led to thoughts, which led to emotions, which eventually led to your behavior.

Identifying My Emotions

Skills Trainer:

Before you learn how to regulate your emotions, you have to learn how to recognize them. As we have discussed, people sometimes react to a situation *based on how they feel, rather than rationally considering how to respond. Similarly, when people are experiencing negative emotions, they may ruminate about how they feel, causing themselves to feel "trapped" in that emotion. Identifying your emotion(s) is the first skill in regulating your emotions and achieving a wise life.*

After you have identified how you feel, it is important to remind yourself that all feelings are temporary. In other words, you may feel sad, or hurt, but that does not mean you will feel sad or hurt forever. One way to manage these negative feelings is to mindfully observe—without judgment—the emotion you are experiencing in the moment. People are less likely to suffer from negative emotions when they can identify the feeling in the moment and say, "I notice I am feeling …" Mindful observation of emotions requires you to identify the various ways in which your emotions manifest themselves. For example, when you are sad or hurt, do you cry? Do you stay in bed all day? Do you think about hurting yourself? What about when you feel hostile toward another person? Do you have a knot in your stomach? Do you clench your fists? Do you think about hurting the other person?

Ask participants to take out Handout 2.2: The Feeling Wheel and Handout 14.2: Ways to Describe Emotions, and explain how an individual's

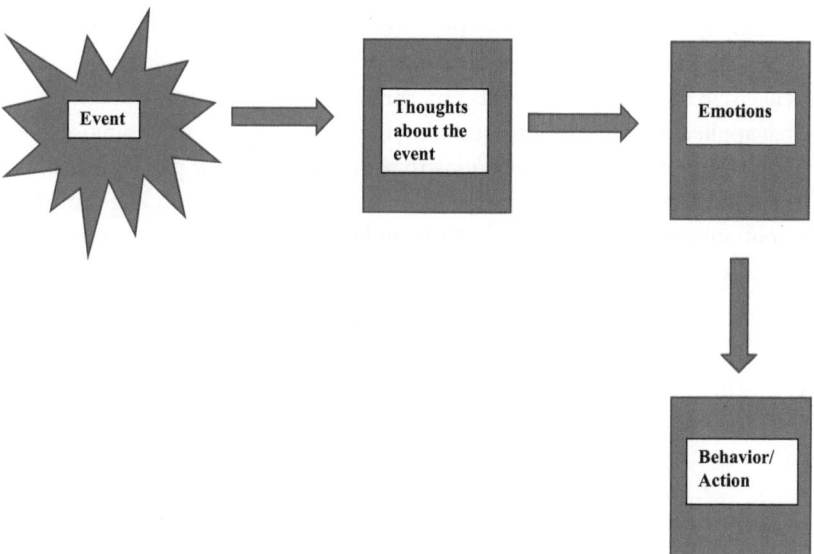

Figure 14.1 Cognitive Behavioral Model

perceptions/interpretations of an event may become intensified depending on their thoughts, emotions, and interpretations of somatic experiences.

> *Loneliness, arousal, and anger are some common emotions that lead men to commit sexual offenses. In order to avoid, disrupt, or change these feelings, it is important to understand common events that prompt the emotion; your interpretation of, or thoughts about, the situation; the bodily sensations that accompany the feeling; and the behavior(s) that follow. This differs from the offense staircase because you are specifically identifying thoughts and feelings associated with your offense, rather than outside circumstances.*

Review Handout 14.2: Ways to Describe Emotions with the group. This handout provides examples of various emotions; possible prompting events leading to the emotion; possible interpretations of the emotion; physiological changes that may occur when feeling the emotion; ways in which the individual may express the emotion; and the aftereffects of the experience. Ask them how identification and descriptions of their emotions may help them to avoid reoffending.

Group Activity: Ask group members to write down two or three emotions other than what is listed in their handout associated with their offense. Ask them to use the cognitive-behavioral model to describe the circumstances leading up to their offense. Discuss participants' responses as a group.

For the homework (Handout 14.2: Ways to Describe Emotions), clients will circle the emotions, events, interpretations, expressions, and aftereffects that applied to them prior to or during the commission of their offense. Next, they will consider other emotions that they experienced prior to or during the offense, and add them to the list, including the corresponding prompting event; interpretation of the emotion; and physiological response, expression, and aftereffects.

Handout 14.1: Myths I Have about Emotions

- Real men don't express their emotions.

  Challenge: _____

- Having emotions means I am not in control of myself.

  Challenge: _____

- When I experience an emotion, I should push it away.

  Challenge: _____

- When I experience an emotion, I should act on it right away.

  Challenge: _____

- Negative emotions are bad.

  Challenge: _____

- I should not allow myself to feel negative emotions.

  Challenge: _____

- I am entitled to express my emotion(s) however I want.

  Challenge: _____

- If I feel a strong emotion, I should express it immediately, regardless of where I am or what I am doing.

  Challenge: _____

- I don't need to manage my emotions because others should be receptive to them.

  Challenge: _____

- My emotions are facts.

  Challenge: _____

- Everyone has ongoing chaos/drama in their lives.

  Challenge: _____

- It is okay to create a little chaos/drama once in a while to make life more interesting.

  Challenge: _____

- I will react however I want because "this is just who I am."

  Challenge: _____

- Emotions happen for no reason.

  Challenge: _____

- Other ideas? _____

  Challenge: _____

Handout 14.2: Ways to Describe Emotions

For this assignment, you will circle the emotions, events, interpretations, expressions, and aftereffects that applied to you prior to or during the commission of your offense. Next, you will consider other emotions that you may have experienced prior to or during the offense, and add them to the list. Don't forget to include the corresponding prompting event; interpretation of the emotion; and the physiological response, expression, and aftereffects.

Ways to Describe Loneliness				
Rejected	Outcast	Isolated	Reclusive	Abandoned
Alone	Withdrawn	Lonesome	Empty	Unattached
Secluded	Disconnected	Neglected	Separate	Dissociated

Prompting Events for Feeling Loneliness				
Getting dumped	Losing a job	Roommate moving	Not being able to attend family events	Other?
Someone passing away	Being ignored by partner/ spouse	Staying home all day	Losing certain freedoms due to probation	
Not having close friends	Children leaving the home	Going to jail	Having an argument with a loved one	

Interpretations of Events that Prompt Feelings of Loneliness

Believing you are a victim	Believing you will always feel lonely	Blaming others	Telling yourself you deserve to feel this way because you are a bad person	Other?
Telling yourself you are a "loser"	Believing you are being punished	Believing you will never find a partner	Telling yourself you "should" feel differently	
Telling yourself "I deserve X to feel better"	Allowing yourself to ruminate about how badly you feel	Telling yourself that people don't like you because …	Isolating yourself at home	

Physiological Changes and Experiences of Loneliness

Knot in stomach	Exhaustion	Becoming sexually aroused	Other?
Urge to cry	Increased heartbeat	Numbness in parts of the body	

Expressions and Actions of Loneliness

Viewing pornography	Exposing yourself in public	Hanging out with friends who don't make good life choices	Skipping work	Binge drinking/or drug use
Going out to find someone to "hook up" with	"Peeping" on others without consent	Sleeping for long periods of time	Canceling obligations	Other?
Masturbating	Going to a strip club	Engaging in self-sabotage behavior	Overeating	

Aftereffects of Loneliness			
Feeling disgust with yourself	Losing relationships	Feeling sad	Other?
Dissociating	Feeling sorry for yourself	Ongoing drug or alcohol use/abuse	
Losing a job	Continued isolation	Going to jail	

Ways to Describe Feeling Aroused			
Sexual	Squirrelly	Lustful	Excited
Giddy	On fire	Passionate	Erotic
Stimulated	Sexy	Hot	

Prompting Events for Feeling Aroused				
Have not had sex in a while	Feeling depressed	Using drugs or alcohol	Running into an ex-partner	Other?
Feeling lonely	Feeling anxious	Seeing an attractive person	Waking up with an erection	
Feeling bored	Meeting a potential sexual partner	Talking to friends about sex	Completing a task·	

Interpretations of Events Prompting Feeling Aroused				
"I need to have sex/ masturbate now!"	"If I just had a partner, I wouldn't feel this way."	"I deserve to have sex/ masturbate to reward myself".	"Children are sexual beings and need to learn somehow ..."	"She's dressed like that, so she obviously wants it."
"I need to watch pornography."	"I can't help it. I'm just addicted to sex."	"I will feel better if I just ..."	"Men are just wired this way."	
"My partner isn't giving me enough sex."	"People who won't have sex with me are losers."	"I need to find someone to hook up with now!"	"Age is just a number."	

Physiological Changes and Experiences of Feeling Aroused			
Erection	Feeling anxious	Feeling warmer	Other?
Heart beating faster	Feeling excited	Skin flushes	

Expressions and Actions of Feeling Aroused				
Looking for someone online to hook up with	Viewing pornography/ having sexual fantasies	Rubbing/ touching a stranger for sexual pleasure	Going to a strip club	Other?
Going to a bar to meet someone to hook up with.	Going to a public place to look at children	Grooming children	Making obscene phone calls	
Masturbating	Exposing yourself/ masturbating in public	Looking for a prostitute	Touching an animal's genitals	

Aftereffects of Feeling Aroused			
Feeling disgusted	Feeling shame	Feeling confused	Other?
Withdrawing from others	Feeling relieved	Decrease of self-esteem	
Feeling guilt	Feeling satisfied	Feeling powerful	

Anger Words			
Aggravated	Agitated	Furious	Annoyed
Frustrated	Rage	Hostility	Vengeful
Grumpy	Irritated	Enraged	Bitter

Prompting Events for Feeling Anger		
Being rejected	Not getting what you want	Other?
Losing a job	Physical pain	
Being criticized		

Interpretations of Events that Prompt Feelings of Anger				
"I deserve …"	"That person deserves … for treating me this way."	"She's promiscuous, so she owes me sex."	"My feelings are the only feelings that matter."	Ruminating about the event that made you angry.
"Women owe men …"	Believing you are right and others are wrong.	"The law doesn't apply to me."	"Everyone just misunderstands me."	Believing people are trying to sabotage you.
"Women are there for men's pleasure."	"Women play mind games."	"I can do whatever I want."	Blaming others.	Other?

Physiological Changes and Experiences of Anger			
Clenching hands	Muscles tensing	Feeling like hitting someone/ something	Feeling "trapped" in the situation
Feeling hot flashes	Knot in stomach	Feeling like you are going to explode	Feeling aroused
Jaw tightening	Face gets flushed	Feeling like crying/crying	Other?

Expressions and Actions of Anger				
Shutting down	Throwing things	Calling names	Making threats	Making impulsive decisions
Being defensive	Hitting someone/ something	Being sarcastic	Sexual offending	Being passive-aggressive
Walking away	Verbally or emotionally attacking someone	Criticizing others	Drinking/ using drugs	Other?

Aftereffects of Anger			
Continued rumination about the situation	Narrowing of attention (having "blinders")	Creating a narrative about the other person	Other?
Dissociating/ feelings of numbness	Feelings of shame	Exhaustion	
Feelings of guilt/ regret	Thinking about what you would do to the person "next time"	Loss of friends/ family	

Note

1 Galietta & Rosenfield (2012).

References

Galietta M., & Rosenfeld B. (2012). Adapting dialectical behavior therapy (DBT) for the treatment of psychopathy. *International Journal of Forensic Mental Health, 11*(4), 325–335.

Changing My Emotional Responses and Conditioning Wise Mind

15

Skills Trainer: Summarize last week:

Thoughts about an event drive our feelings, and ultimately influence how we choose to respond—or react. Have you ever been told, "Just think positively and you'll feel better," or "Just remind yourself how good your life is compared to others"? We refer to this as "toxic positivity." It is frustrating hearing people say these things—especially if you cannot seem to pull yourself out of your depression, soothe your anxiety, or stop feeling that knot in your stomach every time you leave the house. When people respond to your experiences with toxic positivity, it feels as though your experiences and feelings are being invalidated.

You might be wondering, "But how do I make myself feel better when I'm in this terrible situation?" The answer is: you have the ability to "rewire" your brain to reduce the frequency, intensity, and duration of negative emotions. Although you may not be able to attain immediate happiness in the moment— particularly after experiencing a negative event—you can use various skills to regulate the impact of your emotions on yourself and others, and avoid further suffering. Here are some options you can choose to try:

- *Change your emotional response to the problem.*
- *Solve the problem.*
- *Accept the situation (radical acceptance).*
- *Stay upset, or make the situation worse.*

Explain that there are three ways that we can change our emotional responses to a potentially upsetting event: checking the facts; doing an "opposite

DOI: 10.4324/9781003451099-20

action"; and problem solving. Tell clients that it is important to recognize when they are having an intense emotion. When this happens, encourage clients to pause and ask themselves the following questions:

• "Is this thought helpful?"
• "Is this thought a fact?"
• "Would others in the same position likely feel exactly how I feel??

Ask clients to look at Handout 15.1: How to Fact Check. Review it with them using the following example (or an example of your choice):

> Brian and his partner have not been getting along well. It has been five weeks since they have had any sexual activity together, so Brian makes a romantic gesture. He has cooked dinner, bought flowers, and lit candles to create a romantic ambiance in hopes that his partner will want to have sex later on. When his partner arrives home, they are in a bad mood because they got in an argument with a coworker. They ignore the romantic gestures, and say, "I'm going to bed." Brian becomes enraged.

Ask participants how they can help Brian fact check his emotional response to the situation. Ask them to provide examples using the format in Handout 15.1: How to Fact Check.

Skills Trainer: Review Handout 15.2: Emotions that Fit the Facts. Ask group members to split up into small groups of three. Each group will be given three emotions and asked to create examples of situations where the facts fit the emotions. Once each small group has completed the activity, everyone will come back together as a large group and share their scenarios and corresponding emotions. You may notice clients present scenarios where the emotions do not fit the facts. At the end of each list of scenarios for a given emotion, ask the entire group to provide feedback.

Opposite Action

Skills Trainer:
Have you ever heard the saying, "Fake it 'til you make it?" Our emotional responses have corresponding action urges; however, sometimes people's action urges are unhealthy, unhelpful, ineffective, or illegal. Another way of regulating emotions is by doing the opposite of what your body is telling you to do in the moment. In other words, you take an opposite action to "trick" your body and mind until the emotion changes.

Review Handout 15.3: Taking Opposite Action with the group, and discuss the examples listed below. Next, explain the steps to take to create an opposite action and counter an intense, painful emotion.

Ask group members to get back into their small groups of three. Each small group will be asked to come up with urges they feel and possible opposite actions when they experience the emotions they were assigned earlier. Once each small group has completed the activity, everyone will come back together as a large group and share their responses. Again, ask the entire group to provide feedback.

Examples of Opposite Actions		
Emotion	Action/urge	Opposite action
Loneliness	• Isolate • Have sex with a person you do not know • Masturbate	• Call a friend/loved one to talk or get together • Continue trying to meet people when you go out • Join a MeetUp group • Physical activity • Change your posture
Arousal	• Watch pornography • Chat with people online to find someone to "hook up" with • Masturbate • Expose genitals in public	• Take a cold shower • Smell ammonia salts • Snap a rubber band on your wrist • Go for a walk/run/bike ride • Rub ice on your wrists • Practice mindfulness
Anger	• Yell/scream at someone • Attack someone or • something • Punch the wall • Use drugs or alcohol	• Smile • Relax your body. Do a body scan and/or deep breathing • Listen to/sing an upbeat song • Dance • Call someone and tell them something you appreciate/love about them
Love		

Sadness		
Guilt		
Shame		
Happiness		
Fear		
Jealousy		
Anxiety		
Frustration		

Problem-Solving Skills

Skills Trainer:

You have probably been told to use your "problem-solving skills" before, but you may have wondered what these actually look like in practice. There are two ways you can respond to a problem. First, you can choose to avoid the problem and walk away. Avoidance can be helpful or unhelpful, depending on the situation. For example, walking away or avoiding a situation can be problematic when you have a disagreement with your partner and use the stonewalling technique instead of using wise mind and discussing the problem. An example of using wise mind to avoid a situation might include being verbally attacked or harassed at some point in prison and walking away from the other person. Did you walk away from the person yelling at you or calling you names? If so, it was probably because you did not want the situation to escalate and turn into violence.

Your second option is to address a problem head-on. "Addressing the problem" does not refer to you fighting with another person. In other words, sticking around to fight with the person provoking you would probably lead to you getting sent to solitary confinement. Using this example, avoidance is probably the best tactic. However, in your day-to-day life, you will interact with frustrating people, and encounter situations that must be faced assertively. "Addressing a problem" means asserting yourself in a respectful way that does not compromise your integrity. For example, your employer does not give you a raise after a year despite receiving positive evaluations, because you are on the sex offender registry. There are several steps you may want to consider in addressing this situation. First, before taking any action, review your employer's policies and procedures regarding raises, promotions, and employee evaluations. Familiarize yourself with any relevant laws or regulations that might pertain to your situation.

Second, request a private meeting with your immediate supervisor or HR representative to discuss your performance and compensation. Be respectful and professional when making this request.

Third, during the meeting, present your case for a raise calmly and confidently. Highlight your achievements, positive evaluations, and any additional responsibilities you have taken on since your last evaluation. If possible, you may want to mention specific instances where your performance has exceeded expectations.

Fourth, in a respectful manner, ask your employer to provide specific feedback on why you did not receive a raise despite positive evaluations.

Be prepared for your employer to bring up your status on the sex offender registry. Respond to this concern by explaining any rehabilitation efforts you have made since the offense and explain that your registration does not impact your current job performance.

Fifth, be open to discussing potential solutions such as a performance improvement plan or further opportunities to prove your worth to your employer. Express your commitment to your job and your desire to advance in your career. If possible, agree on a timeframe within which you can expect a decision from your employer or a follow-up meeting. If your employer remains unwilling to provide a raise or address your concerns, you may need to explore other career opportunities or seek legal advice if you believe your treatment is discriminatory or unjust.

Ask clients to take out Handout 15.4: Problem-Solving Steps and review it with them.

Moving Away from Emotion Mind: Conditioning Wise Mind

Skills Trainer:

Recall that a few weeks ago, we discussed how thoughts, emotions, and behaviors can be conditioned. We specifically focused on how unhealthy or unhelpful emotions become conditioned, and lead to unhealthy or illegal behavior. This week, we will learn skills to reduce vulnerability to emotion mind, and begin to condition wise mind. The aim is to practice skills that will, over time, decrease the frequency of emotion mind, and decrease the likelihood that emotion mind will lead you to making illegal, unhealthy, or ineffective decisions.

Ask group members what they think they can do to begin conditioning wise mind and write down their ideas.

Next, ask them to look at Handouts 15.5: Extreme Emotions and 15.6: DAPPER Skills, and explain how these skills reduce vulnerability to emotion mind.

- **Develop positive emotions:** It is important for people to develop positive emotions about general, daily activities. This does not mean that they have to be happy about everything all the time. Rather, we encourage clients to notice—with intention—when they feel content at different times throughout the day and pause to acknowledge the positive feelings. The idea is to condition clients to notice and appreciate "the small stuff" in life. In other words, happiness is not a destination, but rather something we can choose to experience at different times in our lives. Over the last few decades, research has shown that positive emotions trigger the "motivation" and "reward" pathways in our brains. The more frequently we activate this region of the brain (e.g., acknowledging positive moments regularly throughout the day, as fleeting as they may be), the more an individual's brain becomes conditioned to continue to acknowledge positive experiences that lead to an increase in positive emotions, and thus health and mental health benefits.[1] Encourage clients to practice this by pausing for a few seconds once or twice per day when they notice they feel content. Once they can do this, ask them to increase the number of times they pause and reflect throughout each day.

- **Anticipate emotional situations:** Considering and planning for an emotional scenario is helpful to do *before* the situation arises—if it ever does—to ensure people have coping strategies in place, so they do not "freeze" or resort to impulsive behaviors in the moment. Encourage clients to review Handout 15.5: Extreme Emotions and consider adding more potentially emotional scenarios and solutions.

- **Practice doing things that make you feel competent:** Remind clients that they all have skills they are good at. Encourage them to review Handout 2.1: A Life More Worth Living and practice using one or two of the strengths they listed during the week. Creating a daily routine that incorporates one's strengths not only improves that strength, but also gives people a sense of accomplishment.

- **Physical illness and Exercise, and eating balanced meals:** We all know that prison food and medical care are not what they could be. While many of your clients may have had pre-existing conditions prior to prison, these conditions may have been exacerbated by, or may have developed during, their incarceration. A lack of continuity of care when transitioning from prison to the community creates more problems for individuals who struggle with health-related concerns, as they often have difficulty accessing nutritious meals, medical care, or spaces where they can exercise. Common health issues we notice in clients include obesity, high blood pressure, cardiovascular problems, and diabetes. While these conditions may not be curable, they are manageable. It is important that clients consider their health as being part of a life worth living. After all, when you feel sick or struggle with medical symptoms, it is hard to enjoy life. Clients are encouraged to work with their individual therapists and possibly their probation officers to determine how they can begin to consider a healthier lifestyle despite their legal and financial restrictions.

- **Rest:** Lack of sleep has been linked to an array of health and mental health problems, such as cardiovascular disease,[2] type 2 diabetes,[3] obesity,[4] irritability, and mood disorders and anxiety.[5]

Once you have reviewed Handout 15.6: DAPPER Skills, ask clients to consider which skills they think would be useful, and what this would look like in practice. Make sure they describe their thoughts in detail.

Handout 15.1: How to Fact Check

- Identify the emotion you are feeling:
  - Describe how you know this is the emotion you are feeling (i.e., what do you notice in your body?).
- Ask yourself what event prompted this emotion:
  - Describe *only the facts* surrounding the event.
- Ask yourself what your interpretations, assumptions, and thoughts are about the event:
  - Identify other possible interpretations.
  - Consider other points of view.
- Ask yourself if you are assuming a threat is imminent:
  - Identify the threat.
  - Assess the likelihood that the threat will actually happen.
  - Consider other possible outcomes.
- Ask yourself if the situation is a catastrophe:
  - Visualize the catastrophe happening.
  - Visualize coping with the catastrophe by using radical acceptance or problem-solving skills.
- Ask yourself if the emotion or the intensity of the emotion fits the facts you have described above. Are you using your wise mind? If not, how might you better use your wise mind to regulate the intensity of the emotion?

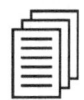

Handout 15.2: Emotions that Fit the Facts

Emotions	Fit the facts
Loneliness	• Breaking up with a partner • Someone you love passes away • You do not have close friends
Arousal	• You have not had sex or masturbated in several days or weeks • Waking up with an erection • Kissing/touching your partner • Fantasizing about your partner
Anger	• You or your loved one is insulted or threatened by someone • You or your loved one is hurt by someone • Being forced to do something you do not feel comfortable doing
Love	
Sadness	
Guilt	
Shame	

Happiness	
Fear	
Jealousy	
Anxiety	
Frustration	

Handout 15.3: Taking Opposite Action

- Identify the emotion you want to change.
- Fact check: Does the emotion fit the situation?
- Describe your urges in the moment.
- Ask wise mind if acting upon your urges would be effective.
- Describe possible opposite actions.
- Act opposite to your urges.

Continue doing this until you notice your emotion change.

Examples of Opposite Actions		
Emotion	**Action/urge**	**Opposite action**
Loneliness	• Isolate • Have sex with a person you do not know • Masturbate	• Call a friend/loved one to talk or get together • Continue trying to meet people when you go out • Join a MeetUp group • Physical activity • Change your posture
Arousal	• Watch pornography • Chat with people online to find someone to "hook up" with • Masturbate • Expose genitals in public	• Take a cold shower • Smell ammonia salts • Snap a rubber band on your wrist • Go for a walk/run/bike ride • Rub ice on your wrists • Practice mindfulness
Anger	• Yell/scream at someone • Attack someone or something • Punch the wall • Use drugs or alcohol	• Smile • Relax your body. Do a body • scan and/or deep breathing • Listen to/sing an upbeat song • Dance • Call someone and tell them something you appreciate/love about them

Love		
Sadness		
Guilt		
Shame		
Happiness		
Fear		
Jealousy		
Anxiety		
Frustration		

Handout 15.4: Problem-Solving Steps

- **Step 1:** Describe the problematic situation.
- **Step 2:** List only the *facts* about the situation. Are you inserting personal thoughts or emotions into this step? If so, try writing down the concrete facts surrounding the situation (e.g., "She said, … Then I said, …").
- **Step 3:** Identify your desired outcome in solving the problem. Is this a realistic outcome? If not, consider outcomes that include compromise (e.g., "I do not want to go back to prison," or "I do not want to lose this relationship").
- **Step 4:** Develop all possible solutions. Are these solutions feasible? Are you willing to try them? Do not include solutions that are not feasible. Be open to trying something new!
- **Step 5:** Choose a solution you believe will help solve the problem, and lead to your desired outcome (or at least a compromise). Which solution do you think will work best to address the problem? Why?
- **Step 6:** Implement your solution. Put your solution into action!
- **Step 7:** Assess the results of your action. Did your solution work? If not, go back to Step 5 and try the next best solution on your list.

Handout 15.5: Extreme Emotions

Come up with two examples of times when you experienced extreme emotions that led to unhealthy/illegal behavior. List the possible solutions you could have considered instead.

Extreme emotion leading to problematic behavior	Possible solutions
	1. 2. 3. 4.
	1. 2. 3. 4.

Now, think about three potential events that could lead to you getting stuck in emotion mind. Try to anticipate potentially problematic scenarios, and come up with solution ideas.

Potentially problematic scenarios	Solutions

Handout 15.6: DAPPER Skills

Skill	How to do it
Develop positive emotions	• Practice doing opposite actions. • Keep track of personal "small • victories"; use progress you have • already made as "evidence" to support that your efforts do pay off.
Anticipate emotional situations	• Plan ahead! Go back to Handout 15.5: Extreme Emotions to view your list of possible solutions.
Practice doing things that make you feel competent	• Go back to Handout 2.1: A Life More Worth Living, and practice, especially when you are "in a rut." • Increase doing (legal and healthy) things that make you happy. • Be mindful! Fully engage in the event.
Physical illness—treat physical ailments	• If you have an injury or illness, seek medical attention right away, to avoid it getting worse. • Drink plenty of water—dehydration contributes to many physical ailments. • Take only the recommended/prescribed dose of over-the-counter or prescription medications.
Exercise and eat balanced meals	• Begin by taking short walks a few times per week. Increase the length, intensity, and/or frequency of your exercise each week. • Limit foods which aren't healthy for your body, such as fried foods and foods high in sugar. • Make sure to eat fruits, vegetables, and "healthy fats" (avocados, nuts); and rely on protein to keep you feeling full. • Drink enough water every day.
Rest	• Aim to get at least seven to nine hours of uninterrupted sleep per night. • Create a sleep schedule: wake up and go to bed around the same time each day. • Practice good sleep hygiene: at least an hour before bedtime, cut off exposure to TV screens, bright lights, and highly stimulating activities.

Handout 15.7: Emotions I Want to Change

This week, you will keep track of your recurring unhelpful emotions, and how you apply skills to address them:

- Write down the emotions you experience this week.
- Consider the various skills you have learned. Which skills, if any, did you use? Be sure to keep track of the contexts/situations in which they arise, and their intensity throughout the week.

It is possible that some of the skills you practiced were not helpful. In this case, go back through the handouts and choose other skills that might be more helpful.

Emotion	Emotional intensity (1–10, where 10 is most extreme)	Context/ situation	Skills I will use to decrease the intensity	Emotional intensity after I use my skills

Notes

1 Cohn, Fredrickson, Brown, Mikels, & Conway (2009); Kok, Coffey, Cohn, Catalino, Vacharkulksemsuk, & Algoe (2013).
2 American Heart Association (2015).
3 Shan, Ma, Xie, Yan, Guo, Bao, & Liu (2015).
4 Wu, Zhai, & Zhang (2014).
5 Division of Sleep Medicine at Harvard Medical School (2007); Gold & Sylvia (2016).

References

American Heart Association. (2015). *Sleep Apnea and Heart Disease, Stroke.* https://www.heart.org/en/health-topics/sleep-disorders/sleep-apnea-and-heart-disease-stroke

Cohn, M. A., Fredrickson, B. L, Brown, S. L., Mikels, J. A., Conway, A. M. (2009). Happiness unpacked: Positive emotions increase life satisfaction by building resilience. *Emotion, 9(3):* 361–368. https://doi.org/10.1037/a001952

Gold, A. K., & Sylvia, L. G. (2016). The role of sleep in bipolar disorder. *Nature and Science of Sleep, 8,* 207–214. https://doi.org/10.2147/NSS.S85754

Kok, B. D., Coffey, K. A., Cohn, M. A., Catalino, L. I., Vacharkulksemsuk, T., Algoe, S. B. (2013). How positive emotions build physical health: Perceived positive social connections account for the upward spiral between positive emotions and vagal tone. *Psychological Science, 24,* 1123–1132. https://doi.org/10.1177/0956797612470827.

Shan, Z., Ma, H., Xie, M., Yan, P., Guo, Y., Bao, W., & Liu, L. (2015). Sleep duration and risk of type 2 diabetes: A meta-analysis of prospective studies. *Diabetes Care, 38(3),* 529–537. https://doi.org/10.2337/dc14-2073

Wu, Y., Zhai, L., & Zhang, D. (2014). Sleep duration and obesity among adults: A meta-analysis of prospective studies. *Sleep Medicine, 15(12),* 1456–1462. https://doi.org/10.1016/j.sleep.2014.07.018

Part V
Distress Tolerance Skills

Coping Ahead   **16**

STOP and CABB Skills

Preparing for Emotional Situations

Skills Trainer: The purpose of coping ahead skills is to work with clients to consider the possibility of emotional situations that could arise in the future.

Improving self-confidence is one way to avoid potentially negative situations, and thus emotional collapse. It is also a protective factor against depression and anxiety.[1] Improving self-confidence, however, is easier said than done. You can't just snap your fingers and feel confident; confidence requires mastery of skills. Mastering skills takes time. Think of your brain as a muscle. When you want to increase the size of your muscles, you have to increase the amount of weight you lift; but you can't just immediately add an additional 50 pounds to your workout regimen. Let's say you can squat 50 pounds, and you want to squat 150 pounds. You wouldn't just add 100 pounds and begin squatting the desired weight; rather, you have to increase the weight slowly. During your first week of training, you may add five or 10 pounds and practice fewer repetitions than usual, to get your body accustomed to the new weight. The following week, you might stay at the same weight but increase the number of repetitions. You will do this until you can increase the weight again, and so on. We master life skills the same way we master anything else—through daily practice. When we master life skills, we are better prepared for whatever curveballs life might throw at us.

DOI: 10.4324/9781003451099-22

Group Discussion: Ask group members to share about a time when they wanted to gain mastery over something in their life (e.g., building something, obtaining a degree or certification, getting better at a sport, exercising), and accomplished their goal. Ask them to share all of the steps involved in mastering their goal. Be mindful that some clients may not have mastered anything because they have not had the desire to do so; or may have a tendency to quit in the middle of projects or activities. In this case, ask them about something they would like to accomplish, and what steps are involved in mastering it.

Common themes that emerge from this discussion are likely that each person felt unsure of themselves at first; they were fearful of failure; they had to continuously work at mastering their skill and not give up; and they gained confidence.

> **Skills Trainer:**
> *Now, you may be wondering what building mastery has to do with coping ahead. "Coping ahead" involves visualizing a problematic situation that could arise in the future, and planning how to address it before it happens.*

Ask clients to imagine a real-life situation that would likely make them react using emotion mind, rather than respond with wise mind. The situation could be something they have already encountered or something that is likely to occur. Once they have visualized the situation, ask them to write it in the "Problem Situation #1" box on Handout 16.1: Building Mastery and Coping Ahead. Next, ask them to write, in detail, how they envision coping with the situation legally and effectively. Finally, explain that there are skills that require mastery in order to cope ahead. Clients should write down what skills they think they need to master in order to cope ahead.

Roleplay: Ask clients to split into groups of two. This is their opportunity to practice coping ahead and determine whether the solutions to their potential problems are effective or need adjustment. One person (Partner A) will act out their partner's problem situation. Their partner (Partner B) will then rehearse the solution out loud. Person A will then slightly increase the intensity of the problem (i.e., "poke the bear") in order to push Person B to think about strategies they may not have considered initially.

> *An example might include the following scenario: James (Partner A) and Connor (Partner B) are neighbors. Connor encounters James while taking a walk, and James says, "Hey, I looked you up, and you're a registered sex offender! Stay away from my kids. I'm going to be watching you from now*

on." Connor practices coping ahead by ignoring the comment and walking away. Ignoring and walking away from potentially problematic or dangerous situations can be very effective, but only if the other person lets go of the issue.

Let's say James then follows Connor and says, "Child molesters don't deserve to live outside of prison. You'd better stay inside your house. If I see you walking around, we're going to have problems." In this situation, James has provoked the situation. Connor may consider adjusting his response slightly.

At this point in the scenario, Partner B will then share how he felt as he was placed in a more intense situation. Partner A and one of the skills trainers should provide Person B with feedback.

Homework: For their homework, participants will practice visualizing a different scenario and complete the exercise on Handout 16.1: Building Mastery and Coping Ahead. Participants are welcome to add more problem situations if they wish. They should begin practicing mastery of their skills each day. Encourage them to keep track of their practice on their diary card.

STOP and CABB Skills

Skills Trainer:
We have learned skills to regulate our emotions. But what happens if you find yourself in a particularly distressing situation or crisis? When people face crises, they go into "fight-or-flight" mode. At times such as these, fixating on the emotion leads to a negative outcome. The purpose of learning distress tolerance skills is to help us survive an immediate crisis without increasing our suffering. These skills should not be used as long-term coping skills, because they are only meant to help when we are faced with immediate threats. In other words, these skills are not likely to make you feel better in the long run, but rather to help you cope with the moment by "doing what works." Then, once the intense, immediate emotion decreases, you will proceed to use your emotion regulation skills.

Note: Highlight the difference immediate threats (e.g., getting hit by a car), and immediate risky situations (e.g., feeling the urge to touch your stepdaughter).

Group Discussion: Ask clients to come up with examples of crisis situations/immediate threats they have experienced (e.g., an attack or anticipated attack in prison; a strong urge to touch a child; suicidal thoughts) and write them on the whiteboard. Next, ask each group member to identify the feeling associated with the threat and how they responded to it. Ask them if their response was both helpful and effective.

STOP Skills

> **Skill Trainer:** Ask participants to take out Handout 16.2: STOP Skills. Explain that they have made some decisions in their past that were neither helpful nor effective; and that despite how difficult it might be to avoid acting on their urges, there are skills that can help them in future situations.
>
> *The skills we are going to learn are the STOP skills: "Stop," "Take a step back," "Observe," and "Proceed mindfully."*

- *__Stop__: Stop what you are doing when faced with an immediate threat; do not react to the real or perceived threat because you want to address it effectively for your own wellbeing.*
- *__Take a step back__: This means detaching yourself from the situation momentarily. Whether we have conditioned our own reaction in these situations, or have never experienced the situation, our mind tends to shift to "autopilot" and react to an intense emotion/perceived crisis. Take deep breaths until the extreme emotion begins to decrease.*
- *__Observe__: Notice what is going on around you. Recall the second group session where we learned about the what skills. Stopping, taking a step back, and observing help us avoid jumping to conclusions and reacting in a way that might cause us problems. In order to address the situation in an effective way, observe what is happening around you and inside your body in the moment. Consider the relevant facts about the moment.*
- *__Proceed mindfully__: When we are faced with a crisis, our emotions become heightened and we tend to feel helpless. When this happens, we are in emotion mind, which increases our risk of making ineffective and even detrimental decisions. Once you have observed your internal feelings and sensations, the external facts about the situation, and your own discomfort, ask yourself what using wise mind would look like. Ask yourself, "How can I proceed mindfully without making things worse?" Now, let's take a look at what the STOP skills might look like in practice.*

Example: Mark is walking down an aisle at the grocery store and notices an unsupervised child walking toward him, looking for her mother. The child looks like she is around age 10, Mark's age preference. She is wearing tight pants and a tight shirt, and Mark finds her very attractive. Mark pauses to look at the child and quickly becomes aroused. He has the urge to walk up to the child, make conversation with her, and touch her crotch. Mark is experiencing an immediate disaster scenario. How can he use the STOP skills to avoid placing himself and the child in danger?

At this point, the skills trainer will stop and ask the group how Mark should use the STOP skills to address this situation. If participants are having trouble applying the skills to the scenario, you can help them.

- <u>*S*</u>: *Mark should stop where he is. He should not proceed walking toward the child.*
- <u>*T*</u>: *Next, Mark could take a few deep breaths to help him decrease his rapid heart rate, and arousal level.*
- <u>*O*</u>: *Mark observes what is happening inside and around him. He notices that his heart is beating rapidly, and his penis is becoming erect. He further notices that he finds the child attractive, and that their parent is not supervising them at that moment.*
- <u>*P*</u>: *Mark has an urge to walk up to the child and use grooming behaviors to make physical contact with them. Mark recognizes his intense urge to have contact with the child, but remembers that he is currently on probation and is registered on the Sex Offender Registry. He uses his wise mind to remind himself that his attraction to children has gotten him in serious trouble in the past, and that despite his urge to offend, he must walk away.*

Mark has safely and effectively managed the crisis situation, but he continues to think about the child throughout the day. Every time he thinks about the child, his heart begins to race and he begins to feel aroused. Mark has removed himself from the dangerous situation. It is now necessary for Mark to use his emotion regulation skills to address his intense lingering emotions about the encounter.

Group Discussion: Ask clients to think of different scenarios where they would be wise to weigh the pros and cons before responding to the threat. In order to do this, it is important to:

- Describe the crisis behavior they want to stop.
- Consider the advantages and disadvantages of acting on their urge.
- Consider the long-term and short-term consequences of acting on the urge.
- Weigh the pros and cons of acting on the behavior.

Clients may have trouble identifying crisis behaviors. If this is the case, provide them with a possible example, such as:

> *You and your stepdaughter are the only people at home. She is walking around in a tight shirt and short pants. Your urge might be to masturbate, touch her, fantasize about her. What are the advantages and disadvantages of doing one of these behaviors?*

	Pros	Cons
Acting on crisis urge	Advantages	Disadvantages
Resisting crisis urge	Advantages	Disadvantages

Ask group members to share their pros and cons lists. Encourage the other group members to provide feedback. Explain that some people find it helpful to say "NO" out loud, or snap a rubber band on their wrist, to avoid acting on the crisis behavior.

CABB Skills

This week, you will specifically teach your group how to use the CABB skills. In other words, you will explain each of the breathing techniques, and the body scan, and then ask participants to practice as you talk them through these exercises. If you can, you may want to bring in small bowls of ice water and/or ice cubes to practice the cold-water skill. Ask participants to take out Handout 16.3: CABB Skills.

Skills Trainer:
Last week, we learned the STOP skills to tolerate crisis situations. This week, we are learning a new set of skills to manage the physiological arousal that occurs during these situations. There are four CABB skills: "cold water," "aerobic exercise," "breathing with intention," and "body scan."

Physiological arousal occurs when our nervous system is activated. The nervous system is complex and is, in part, responsible for recognizing environmental changes and impacting your bodily responses. Part of the nervous system consists of the sympathetic nervous system, which is responsible for the "fight-or-flight" response to distressing situations. When this response is activated, our parasympathetic nervous system—the part of our nervous system that regulates emotions and bodily functions—becomes less regulated, leading to an increased negative arousal state. Using CABB skills increases the parasympathetic nervous system's ability to come back to equilibrium, or the "rest-and-digest" state.

There are numerous benefits of using CABB skills, such as quickly decreasing negative emotional states; and they work immediately. These skills help to disrupt negative thoughts that could lead to destructive behavior such as destroying property, self-harming, or harming another person. In addition, you can use your CABB skills to re-center yourself and come back to the moment when you are overwhelmed and stuck in emotion mind.

Here is an example of when your CABB skills come in handy. Think back to your sexual regulation skills. What happens if you are masturbating and a thought of your victim, or a specific non-consensual person, pops into your head? No matter how sexually aroused you are, DO NOT ORGASM to the thought! In this scenario, you are highly aroused and, let's face it, you really want to have that orgasm. The first step, however, is to immediately stop masturbating, then use your CABB skills. First, you can shock your nervous system out of your aroused state by using some of the ideas listed on Handout 16.3: CABB Skills, or coming up with other ideas.

Breathing Exercises

Depending on the space, briefly teach participants each breathing exercises while sitting in a chair, on the floor, or lying down. Tell participants the following for the first three breathing techniques:

We will practice each exercise for two minutes. Make yourself comfortable. If you are sitting, straighten your back, lift your shoulders to your ears, and roll them back so you are sitting in an upright position. Place your hands on your thighs, or on your stomach.

- **Box breathing:** *Close your eyes and imagine a square box in front of you. Start at one corner of the box and breathe in through your nose for a count of four. At the next corner of the box, hold your breath and count to four. Again, at the next corner, breathe out through your mouth for a count of four. Finally, at the last corner of box, hold the outbreath for a count of four. Continue to visualize the sides of the box as you breathe and count.*
- **Triangle breathing:** *Close your eyes and imagine a triangle in front of you. Start at the bottom left-hand side of the triangle and breathe in through your nose for three counts. At the top of the triangle, hold your breath for three counts. At the last corner of the triangle, breathe out through your nose for three counts, and hold for three seconds.*
- **Mindful breathing:** *Place your hands on your stomach. Imagine your stomach is a hot air balloon. Take a deep breath in through your nose. Feel your lungs and stomach expand. Now, breathe out slowly through your nose or mouth and feel your lungs and stomach deflate. Your thoughts will begin to wander. When this happens, non-judgmentally notice that your mind has wandered, and bring it back to your breathing.*
- **Lion's breath (modified):** *Sit in a comfortable position on the floor, or on a cushion on the floor. Lean forward slightly, spread your fingers wide, and place them on your knees or on the floor. Take a deep breath through your nose. Now, open your mouth wide, stretch your tongue out and point it downwards. Exhale from your diaphragm and as you do this, make the sound "Ha." Imagine you are ridding your body of unhelpful thoughts and bringing your body back to a resting state. While exhaling, make a "Ha" sound that comes from deep within your abdomen.*

Body Scan

The body scan is a way to self-sooth and release tension from each part of your body. Lie down on your back, rest your hands on your stomach or on the floor, and close your eyes. Take a few deep breaths. Try to stay still while you complete the scan. Focus your attention on your toes. Do not move them; just notice their presence. Can you feel your socks or shoes touching them? Are they hot or cold? Are they tingling? Do they feel "normal"? Hold the feeling of your toes in your awareness, take a deep breath, and move up to your ankles.

Skills Trainer: Repeat the following each time you move up the body: *Notice its/their presence. Hold the feeling of your [body part] in your awareness, take a deep breath, and move up to your ...*

Continue the scan by asking participants to scan the following:

- Lower legs.
- Knees.
- Upper legs.
- Stomach and pelvis.
- Ribs.
- Chest.
- Fingers and hands.
- Arms.
- Shoulders.
- Neck.
- Ears.
- Head.

This process should take approximately 20 minutes. Make sure to remind participants that when their mind starts to wander, they should bring their attention back to the body part being scanned at that moment.

Handout 16.1: Building Mastery and Coping Ahead

Problem situation #1:
Skills I need to master to cope with the problem:
How I imagine coping with the problem effectively (describe in detail; list the steps):

Problem situation #2:

Skills I need to master to cope with the problem:

How I imagine coping with the problem effectively (describe in detail; list the steps):

Handout 16.2: STOP Skills

- **<u>S</u>top:** Stop what you are doing when faced with an immediate threat; do not *react* to the real or perceived threat.
- **<u>T</u>ake a step back:** Detach yourself from the situation momentarily. Take deep breaths until the extreme emotion begins to decrease.
- **<u>O</u>bserve:** Notice what is going on around you. In order to address the situation in an effective way, observe and describe what is happening around you and inside your body in the moment. Consider the relevant facts about the moment.
- **<u>P</u>roceed mindfully:** Once you have observed your internal emotions and sensations, the external facts about the situation, and your own discomfort, ask yourself what using wise mind would look like. How can you proceed mindfully without making things worse?

Handout 16.3: CABB Skills

- **Cold water:**
  - Take a cold shower.
  - Put cold water on your face.
  - Ice your genitals (use an ice pack or bag of frozen vegetables. Avoid placing it directly on your genitals; instead, use a towel to wrap it up, but not so much that you cannot feel the cold).
  - Hold ice cubes in your hand.
  - Rub your inner arms and wrists with ice cubes.
- **Aerobic exercise:**
  - Go for a run outdoors. You can substitute this for a brisk walk; just make sure you raise your heart rate.
  - Go for a bike ride.
  - Do jumping jacks, jump-squats, burpees, or jump rope until you feel your arousal state decrease. As your heart rate increases, think about how angry or frustrated you are. Pairing negative feelings with an action that decreases your arousal state can help you recondition (decrease) your emotional response should these situations arise again.
  - Put on music and dance.
- **Breathing with intention:**
  - **Box breathing:**
    - Breathe in through your nose for four counts.
    - Hold the breath for four counts.
    - Breathe out through your mouth for four counts.
    - Hold for four counts.
    - Repeat!

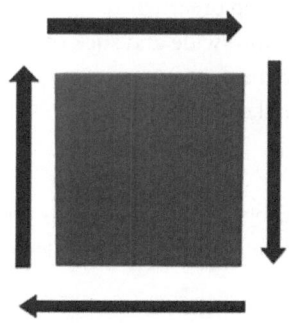

Image 16.1 Box Breathing

- **Triangle breathing:**
  - Breathe in through your nose for three counts.
  - Hold your breath for three counts.
  - Breath out through your nose for three counts.
  - Repeat!

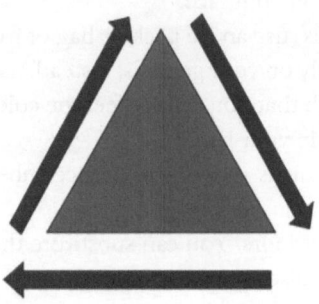

Image 16.2 Triangle breathing

- **Mindful breathing:**
  - Place your hands on your stomach. Take a deep breath in through your nose. Feel your lungs and stomach expand.
  - Breathe out slowly through your nose or mouth and feel your lungs and stomach deflate.
  - Repeat!
- **Lion's breath (modified):**
  - Sit on the floor/on a cushion on the floor.
  - Lean forward slightly.
  - Place your hands on your knees or on the floor.
  - Stretch your fingers.
  - Take a slow, deep breath in.
  - Open your mouth wide and stick out your tongue. Try to make it touch your chin.
  - Exhale and make the sound "Ha."
  - Repeat!
- **<u>B</u>ody Scan:**
  - Lie down on your back, rest your hands on your stomach or on the floor, and close your eyes. Take a few deep breaths.

- Notice the presence of each of the following body parts. In each case, hold the feeling of that body part in your awareness, take a deep breath, and then move your focus on to the next one:
  - Feet.
  - Lower legs.
  - Knees.
  - Upper legs.
  - Stomach and pelvis.
  - Ribs.
  - Chest.
  - Fingers and hands.
  - Arms.
  - Shoulders.
  - Neck.
  - Ears.
  - Head.

Note

1 Diener & Seligman (2002); Dobson (1989).

References

Diener E., & Seligman M. E. P. (2002). Very happy people. *Psychological Science, 13,* 80–83. https://doi.org/10.1111/1467-9280.00415

Dobson K. (1989). A meta-analysis of the efficacy of cognitive therapy for depression. *Journal of Consulting and Clinical Psychology, 57,* 414–419. https://doi.org/10.1037/0022-006X.57.3.414

Self-Soothing, Wise Mind ACCEPTS and RAW PAR Skills

17

Skills Trainer:

Sometimes people experience a distressing situation, and thoughts and memories of that situation continue to pop into their heads throughout the day. These automatic thoughts can be distressing, and can cause the same type of physiological arousal as the original distressing event. You may begin to feel angry; your fists may clench; you may begin to cry or have a headache. Many people have trouble stopping their distressing automatic thoughts, so the thoughts continue to bombard them in the long term. This week, we will learn skills to disrupt those thoughts, self-soothe when they arise, and ultimately accept the thoughts for what they are: just thoughts/memories.

Distracting yourself during a distressing situation helps you decrease your emotional arousal by taking you away from the distressing stimuli and stopping you from engaging in ineffective, potentially harmful behaviors. This does not mean that you disconnect completely from your thoughts, feelings, and sense of identity; rather, it encourages you to temporarily compartmentalize your experience in the moment. Compartmentalizing can be helpful, but it can also be harmful. People tend to compartmentalize in order to move their attention from a distressful situation and focus on something else. However, sometimes people compartmentalize their memories, thoughts, and feelings in such a way that they do not allow themselves the possibility of addressing and processing them at a later time, when they feel less distressed.[1] At this point, compartmentalization can become problematic and create bigger problems in the future.

DOI: 10.4324/9781003451099-23

Group Discussion: Ask participants to think of examples of how they have used compartmentalization in unhealthy or unhelpful ways. Next, ask them to provide an example of when they have used this technique to tolerate a distressing situation.

Then ask participants to think of examples when they experienced intense, distressing emotions, but were unable to address the problems in the moment. Write the responses on the whiteboard and ask participants to write them in their notebooks as well.

> **Skills Trainer:** Ask participants to take out Handout 17.1: Wise Mind ACCEPTS Skills.
>
> *In these instances, there are other skills you can use. This skill set specifically focuses on how to use your wise mind and accept the situation for what it is: radical acceptance. This does not mean that you have to like it, or that you will not experience some discomfort. But you will not experience the same level of discomfort as you would if you did not use your skills. The acronym you are learning today is ACCEPTS, which stands for: "activities," "contributing," "comparisons," "emotions," "pushing away" and "sensations."*
>
> - *__A__ctivities: You can distract yourself and avoid engaging in unhelpful or dangerous behavior by participating in an activity that keeps your mind off the distressing situation. Make sure to have a list of activities you might want to engage in if you are in a situation where you are having trouble thinking about what exactly to do.*
> - *__C__ontributing: This refers to helping another person or people. This could include helping a friend or family member, or volunteering. Research has shown that regularly volunteering helps improve one's overall wellbeing and provides you with a sense of meaning and purpose.[2]*

Note: *Make sure to explain the importance of maintaining healthy boundaries and using self-care. I have found that some men who engage in helping activities tend to overextend their emotional capacity and avoid addressing their own problems. In fact, research on older adults and engagement in volunteering has shown that there is a threshold at which the amount of time spent volunteering begins to diminish one's wellbeing.[3]*

> - *__C__omparisons: Comparing your current situation to previous challenges you have experienced can be helpful to remind yourself that things could be worse than they are right now. This does not mean that your current experience is not distressing or painful, but rather that you have*

experienced more distressing situations and survived them. For example, you may remember the day you were arrested, or spending time in prison. You likely felt scared, sad, and lonely; yet you made it through.

- **Emotions:** You can also distract yourself by eliciting another emotion. This does not happen instantly, or because you will yourself to feel another way. Turn on the TV, listen to music, or read a book or magazine that you know will generate a different, opposite emotion. This can work both in the short term and in the long term. This skill is similar to "opposite action" from the emotion regulation skills module. The difference is that here you are focused on changing your emotion in the moment, specifically to distract yourself from feeling intense distress.

- **Pushing away:** This is similar to briefly compartmentalizing your thoughts about a distressing situation. However, it refers to repeatedly stopping potentially negative behaviors for short periods of time. Over time, the more frequently and the longer you can push these behaviors away, the weaker the urge will become.

  Example: Wallace had a bad day. First, he was fired from his job. Then, when he went home, his partner yelled at him, walked into their bedroom, and slammed the door. Wallace has just experienced two distressing situations, and he knows that masturbating always made him feel better—at least temporarily. So, Wallace decides to use his pushing away skill, and instead of masturbating in that moment, he tells himself that he will delay masturbating until after he makes himself a sandwich. Once he has made the sandwich, he tells himself that he will wait until after he eats the sandwich. Even if Wallace decides to masturbate later that evening, he has delayed the use of sex to cope with a distressing situation.

- **Thoughts:** This involves disrupting your thoughts or distracting yourself with different thoughts. Examples include:
  - Distracting: Some people think of distressing thoughts as clouds sweeping across the sky. Imagine a cloud over your head. Soon, that cloud will float away, because that is what clouds do. Imagine the wind blowing the cloud out of your visual field. Continue using this imagery until you feel you can come back to the present moment.
  - Disrupting: We can disrupt distressing thoughts in a few different ways. For example, you could clap your hands and say "NO" out loud; call a friend or family member; or snap a rubber band on your wrist.

- **Sensations:** Focus on your various sensations.

Skills Trainer: It is helpful to walk clients through each of these exercises:

- *Suck on a candy, or eat a piece of sour candy.*
- *Look around you and try to identify three objects of the same color. Touch two different objects within reach. What do they feel like? Now, pause and listen carefully. Identify two different sounds that you hear within your vicinity. Finally, take a deep breath in through your nose and name two smells around you.*
- *Progressive muscle relaxation:*
  o *Lie down on the floor or find a comfortable reclined position.*
  o *Make sure to loosen tight clothing so you can fully relax.*
  o *Take a few slow, deep breaths.*
  o *Squeeze your feet by curling your toes inward and hold for a count of 20. Take a deep breath in and on your outbreath, relax your feet.*
  o *Squeeze your calf muscles tightly and count to 20. Take a deep breath in and on your outbreath, relax your calves. Notice the stress tension leaving your body.*
  o *Squeeze your hamstrings and quadriceps and hold for 20 seconds. Take a deep breath in and on your outbreath, relax the tension in those muscles.*
  o *Squeeze your buttocks. Hold for 20 seconds. Take a deep breath in and on your outbreath release your muscles.*
  o *Squeeze your stomach muscles as tight as you can. Hold for 20 seconds. Take a deep breath in and on your outbreath, release the muscles. Take an extra few, deep breaths to recenter your breath.*
  o *Make a fist with both hands and tense your biceps. Bring your fists to your chest and hold for 20 seconds, squeezing as tight as you can. Take a deep breath in and on your outbreath, release your muscles, and return your hands to the sides of your body.*
  o *Squeeze your shoulders up toward your ears. Feel the tension in your upper back, and neck. Hold for 20 seconds. Take a deep breath in and on your outbreath, release your muscles. Notice the tension in this area melt away.*
  o *Squeeze the muscles in your face. Make sure to squeeze your lips together tightly. Hold for 20 seconds. Take a deep breath in and on your outbreath, release your muscles.*
  o *Take a few deep breaths and notice the difference in how your muscles feel.*

The body scan and progressive muscle relaxation exercises are particularly helpful when practiced on a daily basis. In fact, over time, this will help you regulate your emotions long term.

Acceptance Skills

Skills Trainer:
Accepting the moment for what it is can be tricky, especially when we desire it to be different. Sometimes people end up stuck in "wanting mind," or wanting a situation or life to be different from what it is in the moment, despite not having the power to change it. This leads to suffering because you are not getting what you want out of the situation, and end up spending an enormous amount of time and effort willing the situation to change. Consider this old analogy, referred to as "letting go of the banana":

Hunters in the tropical forests use a cage and a banana to trap monkeys. They place a banana in the cage, knowing that the monkey will reach into the cage to grab the object of their desire (i.e., the banana). However, the banana is too large to fit through the wires of the cage. The monkey pulls at the banana over and over again, but spends too much focus, time, and energy engaged in grabbing the banana, so the hunters can catch the monkey and place it in the cage. Had the monkey simply let go of the banana, it would have avoided being trapped in the cage.

The take-home message from this analogy is that when we are too focused on a situation or object of desire that we cannot change or have, we get trapped by our own desire, which makes us stuck. This can end up lasting days, months, years, or even a lifetime if we do not practice radical acceptance and accept the moment for what it is, despite not liking it. In other words, let go of the banana!

The purpose of learning acceptance skills is not to eliminate desire for change, per se, but rather to acknowledge one's discomfort, hold it in awareness, and accept it for what it is right now. This week we will learn RAW PAR: six reality acceptance skills (Handout 18.2: RAW PAR Skills) that you can use when you find yourself in wanting mind. They include: "radical acceptance," "allowing the mind," "willingness," "partial smile," "accepting hands," and "refocusing the mind."[4]

- *Radical acceptance: Throughout your treatment, you have learned skills to create change in your life, so it may be confusing that you are now being taught to accept uncomfortable or distressing situations. In other words, you may think that if you accept these situations, you are allowing yourself to become a victim of life; but this is not the case. You may want to think of situations that require radical acceptance as your "ongoing triggers" from Handout 8.1: My Offense Staircase.*

- *Example: Marty is attracted to girls between the ages of 12 and 15. He knows that it is illegal to have sex with a minor, and that doing this has gotten him into trouble in the past. Girls between the ages of 12 and 15 are Marty's desired sexual partners. In fact, he has trouble becoming aroused with adults. Marty likely cannot change whom he is attracted to. His options are to radically accept that this is his situation, and that he can use his skills to manage not reoffending; or he can choose to reoffend, thus harming another child and ending up back in prison.*

- *Example: Here is another example of when using radical acceptance is helpful: you are currently on probation or parole. No one enjoys having someone enforce specific conditions that you are legally required to abide by. Moreover, you know that if you violate your conditions, you could end up going back to jail or prison.*

Now, ask the group what they can do right now to get off probation tomorrow. They will, of course, tell you that there is nothing they can do. Ask, "So if there is nothing you can do right now to get off probation tomorrow, or even next week, even though you want to, what can you do to have a life worth living, despite these constraints?"

Most of the participants will acknowledge that their only option for getting off probation/parole is to accept their situation for what it is and follow the rules laid out in their conditions. You can say, "This does not mean that you have to like the situation you are in; rather, you fully accept your reality for what it is without fighting it or adopting a victim stance."

Note: Some participants may say that they could violate the conditions of their probation, be revoked, and go back to prison, because being on probation is just the same as, or worse than, prison. If this happens ask, "How would that contribute to your goals of creating a wise life?" or "Is there any possibility that this is emotion mind speaking?"

- *Allowing the mind: This refers to being mindful of your current thoughts. This means that you allow yourself to acknowledge what is going on in your mind without judging yourself or the situation. You can use visualization to practice this skill. Picture yourself lying on your back in the grass, or on the beach. You notice clouds passing overhead. As soon as one cloud passes, another comes into view, and so on. Think about your thoughts as passing clouds: you acknowledge the thought without judgment, and you allow it to pass. You do not need to analyze your thoughts or figure out where they are coming from in the moment.*

- **Willingness:** *Go back to Handout 2.5: Stages of Change. At the beginning of treatment, we talked about the various stages of change, and where you saw yourself in terms of change. "Willingness" refers to how ready you are to make the changes you have the power to make. "Willfulness," on the other hand, is when you try to control people and situations that you cannot control—for example, by:[5]*
  - ○ *Avoiding people/situations that need to be addressed.*
  - ○ *Giving up on people/situations that need to be addressed.*
  - ○ *Denying the existence of problems that need to be addressed.*
  - ○ *Holding grudges.*
  - ○ *Making excuses.*
  - ○ *Focusing only on yourself and your needs and wants.*
- *Willingness, on the other hand, involves:*
  - ○ *Responding to a person or situation using wise mind.*
  - ○ *Acknowledging the importance of interconnectedness (i.e., accepting that we are connected to others, and life requires us to acknowledge not only our own wants and needs, but also those of others).*
  - ○ *"Letting go of the banana."*
  - ○ *Trying something new—despite the discomfort—that could aid in self-improvement.*

Group Discussion: Ask the group to provide examples from their lives of willfulness and willingness. Ask them about the aftereffects of their behavior (e.g., "How did that work out for you?")

Skills Trainer:

The remaining three acceptance skills are: "partial smile", "accepting hands", and "refocusing the mind." These skills can be practiced in any setting, at any time of the day or night.

- **Partial smile:** *A partial smile is one tool for acknowledging and accepting reality even if you are unhappy with the situation.*

   Tell participants to relax their face and lips. Ask them to visualize themselves in a situation they do not want to be in. (Perhaps they were called into their probation/parole officer's office or are anxious about a polygraph.) Tell participants to make a fake smile. Ask,

"How does that make your face feel?" Next, tell them to take a deep breath, and relax their faces and lips once again. Finally, tell participants to partially smile. Ask them about the differences in physical sensations, thoughts, and emotions they noticed with each smile. The goal of this exercise is to show your clients that they do not have to pretend to like an unpleasant situation; rather, they can be true to themselves, and acknowledge and accept their discomfort without becoming emotionally dysregulated.

- *Accepting hands: Accepting hands is another way of demonstrating willingness to accept the situation for what it is in the moment.*

   Ask participants to relax their hands and place them on their thighs with their palms facing upward and take a few deep breaths. Alternatively, they can place their hands—palms facing downward—on their stomach, and feel their stomach inflate and deflate with each breath and outbreath.

   Imagine you are trying to start dating again. You and the other person agree to meet at a certain location at a certain time, but they do not show up; nor do they call you to cancel the date. You are rightfully upset by the situation but begin to engage in unhealthy/unhelpful self-talk. You say, "How dare she stand me up? Typical woman—always playing mind games with men." Or you may tell yourself that it is your fault that people do not want to date you. You may tell yourself that you are a loser, or that no woman would want to date someone convicted of a sexual offense. In these instances, pause, take a deep breath and use accepting hands to remind yourself that while the situation is hurtful, disappointing, and upsetting, it will not change. Maybe something happened to your date and they are at the hospital. Perhaps your date decided at the last minute that she did not want to go on the date and "ghosted" you. Either way, this situation is probably not about something you did, but rather something going on with them. If you call or text the other person to "teach them a lesson," you are moving into emotion and risky mind.

- *Refocusing the mind: This refers to disrupting unhelpful/unhealthy and intrusive thoughts. As discussed in the emotion regulation module, the purpose of refocusing techniques is to avoid rumination and keep your thoughts from "spiraling" and making your situation worse. You may want to think of this skill as "changing the channel" on the television. While this is challenging at first, and negative thoughts may continue to pop up, you will notice that the frequency of the thoughts decreases.*

   Example: Nate used to view child pornography and masturbate to it. When he is bored, upset, or sexually aroused, intrusive thoughts about images he viewed pop into his head. Nate has been working hard to avoid the intrusive thoughts, but they continue to come up. Nate wants to disrupt these thoughts, but avoiding the thoughts is not working. In this case, Nate may consider "changing the channel." Here are some techniques Nate can try:

o   *Looking around the room and describing what he sees.*

o   *Remembering what prison was like.*

o   *Thinking about something he is looking forward to.*

Group Discussion: Now, ask the group to share their thoughts about the pros and cons of using RAW PAR skills. Make a list on the whiteboard. Participants should complete the homework section of Handout 17.2: RAW PAR Skills for next week.

Roleplay: Radical acceptance is easier said than done. It takes practice. Ask group members to break up into groups of two. Person A will identify one problem in his life or a potential problem that could arise where he will have to use radical acceptance. Person B will enact that scenario while Person A practices engaging his distress tolerance skills and practices radical acceptance of the situation. Once Person A is finished, Person B will identify a problem from his life, and so on.

Handout 17.1: Wise Mind ACCEPTS

- **Activities:** You can distract yourself and avoid engaging in unhelpful or dangerous behavior by participating in an activity that keeps your mind off the distressing situation. Make sure to have a list of activities you might want to engage in if you are in a situation where you are having trouble thinking about what exactly to do.
- **Contributing:** This refers to helping another person or people. This could include helping a friend or family member, or volunteering. Research has shown that regularly volunteering helps improve one's overall wellbeing and provides you with a sense of meaning and purpose.
- **Comparisons:** Comparing your current situation to previous challenges you have experienced. This does not mean that your current experience is not distressing or painful, but rather that you have experienced more distressing situations and survived them.
- **Emotions:** Eliciting another emotion. Turn on the TV, listen to music, or read a book or magazine that you know will generate a different, opposite emotion. This skill is similar to "opposite action" from the emotion regulation skills module. The difference is that here you are focused on changing your emotion in the moment, specifically to distract yourself from feeling intense distress.
- **Pushing away:** This refers to repeatedly stopping potentially negative behaviors for short periods of time.
- **Sensations:** Focus on your various sensations.

Handout 17.2: RAW PAR Skills

- **Radical acceptance:** Accepting things as they are in the moment. This does not mean you have to like them.
- **Allowing the mind:** Being mindful of your current thoughts. This means that you allow yourself to acknowledge what is going on in your mind without judging yourself or the situation. You can use visualization to practice this skill.
- **Willingness:** Your readiness to make the changes you have the power to make.
- **Partial smile:** Force yourself to smile, even if you don't feel like it.
- **Accepting hands:** This is another way of demonstrating willingness to accept the situation for what it is in the moment. Relax your hands and place them on your thighs with your palms facing upward and take a few deep breaths. You can also place your palms facing downward on your stomach, and feel your stomach inflate and deflate with each inbreath and outbreath.
- **Refocusing the mind:** Disrupting unhelpful/unhealthy and intrusive thoughts to avoid rumination and to keep your thoughts from "spiraling" and making your situation worse.

Homework

Navigating all of the obstacles in our life can be challenging and frustrating. There are some things that we just have to put up with; but there are other things that we can change to make our lives easier—or at least less frustrating. For this activity, you will identify various factors in three key areas: "Things I have to accept"; "Things I have passively accepted"; and "Things I want to change."

Things I can choose to accept: These are various factors that you either have to accept are part of your life or not accept, thus making yourself feel worse (e.g., probation).

1) _____

2) _____

3) _____

4) _____

5) _____

6) _____

7) _____

8) _____

9) _____

10) _____

Things I have passively accepted: These are factors that contribute to your stress and frustration, but that you have accepted because "it's just easier: (e.g., staying in an unhappy relationship).

1) _____

2) _____

3) _____

4) _____

5) _____

6) _____

7) _____

8) _____

9) _____

10) _____

Things I want to change: These are the various parts of your life that you can control and want to change in order to improve your mood and overall wellbeing. These may be things that you have accepted previously, but would like to change now (e.g., getting out of an unhappy relationship).

1) _____

2) _____

3) _____

4) _____

5) _____

6) _____

7) _____

8) _____

9) _____

10) _____

Now that you have identified these various factors, take a look at your "Things I want to change" list and explain what you will actively do to change them. For example:

- I will find a new place to live within the next two months.
- I will stop spending time with friends who are negative influences.
- If I see a child that I am attracted to, I will turn around and walk in the other direction.
- I will decrease my masturbation from five times per week to three times per week.

My plan for change:

_____

_____

_____

_____

_____

_____

_____

_____

_____

_____

Notes

1 The skills trainer may want to use the example of clients who do not believe there is a need to reflect on their offending behavior as unhelpful compartmentalization.
2 See, for example, Binder & Freytag (2013); Yeung, Zhang & Kim (2018).
3 Windsor, Anstey, & Rodgers (2008).
4 RAW PAR skills adapted from Linehan (2015).
5 You can also ask clients to review Handout 7.1: Thinking Errors, as staying "stuck" with their thinking errors is a form of willfulness.

References

Binder M., & Freytag A. (2013). Volunteering, subjective well-being and public policy. *Journal of Economic Psychology, 34,* 97–119. https://doi.org/10.1016/j.joep.2012.11.008

Linehan M. M. (2015). *Skills Training Manual* (2nd ed.). New York: Guilford Press.

Windsor T. D., Anstey K. J., & Rodgers B. (2008). Volunteering and psychological well-being among young-old adults: How much is too much? *The Gerontologist, 48*(1), 59–70.

Yeung J. W., Zhang Z., & Kim T. Y. (2018). Volunteering and health benefits in general adults: cumulative effects and forms. *BMC Public Health, 18*(1), 1–8. https://doi.org/10.1186/s12889-017-4561-8

Dialectical Abstinence, Lapse Prevention, and Sexual Safety Plan

18

Chapter 2 briefly discussed the distinction between the terms "relapse" and "lapse." During this session, it is important to review the differences, and provide clients with an understanding of the dialectics of remaining abstinent from addictive and/or compulsive behaviors that are likely to lead to reoffending (i.e., dynamic acute risk factors). Behaviors such as substance use/abuse, viewing legal pornography, engaging in frequent masturbation or sex with multiple or unknown partners, and going to sex shops to "browse" are all examples of "lapse" behaviors that can lead to a relapse.

Some men who have committed sex crimes are prohibited from viewing pornography, using substances, and attending sex shops while on supervision. In addition, they are discouraged from engaging in unhealthy sexual practices that likely led to their offending. However, clients nearing the end of their probation or parole may struggle with the idea of, or may be ambivalent about, going back to viewing pornography and masturbating to it, and other risky behaviors. Dialectical abstinence addresses relapse of former addictive or compulsive behaviors from both an abstinence and harm reduction perspective. In other words, the end goal of dialectical abstinence is to completely abstain from the unhealthy and/or illegal behavior, so clients do not reoffend. However, this model also acknowledges that lapses may occur during and after treatment.

The challenge here is that clients who fail to plan for a potential lapse typically fail to recognize that a lapse is possible when working toward complete abstinence; and they take longer to return to abstinence because they tend to punish themselves by labeling themselves as "failures," "losers,"

DOI: 10.4324/9781003451099-24

or "broken," and allowing their cognitive distortions to become more deeply entrenched (e.g., "all-or-nothing" thinking).

Addictive or compulsive behaviors often stem from environmental triggers associated with those behaviors. Consequently, an individual may wish to abstain from certain behaviors and may no longer experience the same level of pleasure engaging in these behaviors that they once did. However, specific environmental triggers can persist in eliciting a surge of dopamine in the brain, which can lead to the individual's inclination to become aroused or engage in masturbation. Thus, even if the individual did not initially wish to masturbate, the presence of these environmental triggers may prompt them to contemplate masturbation and ultimately act upon it.[1]

Skills Trainer:

We have learned about emotion mind, reason mind, risky mind, and wise mind. We can also understand addictive and compulsive behaviors by considering these states of mind. For example, when men who have committed sex offenses have a history of substance abuse or compulsive sexual behaviors, there are many triggers that can lead to risky mind, especially if they are experiencing a particularly distressing emotion (i.e., they are in emotion mind).

Risky mind is when you are engaging in behaviors that directly preceded or were related to your offense. For example, you may have committed your offense while under the influence of drugs or alcohol; or you may have been masturbating frequently to fantasies of illegal situations. Go back to your offense staircase to identify your immediate triggers. You may have also thought of more immediate triggers throughout the course of treatment.

When a person has remained abstinent from the addictive or compulsive behavior for a period of time and tells themselves that they are free from their triggers (i.e., that they no longer have to worry about their triggers), they are engaging their reason mind. This is problematic because the person has failed to acknowledge that there is always the possibility of lapse and thus will not have a plan to address a lapse to avoid reoffending in future.

Example: Tyrone used to view excessive adult pornography—until that was no longer arousing, and he began looking for different, more deviant images. Soon, he came across bestiality and child pornography, which he started viewing, and to which he masturbated. Tyrone is nearing the end of his probation and is contemplating whether to go back to viewing adult pornography; after all, he has abstained from it for the last 10 years, so he wonders how viewing legal porn could possibly be a problem. Tyrone has failed to consider the role of adult pornography in his offending.

Emotion mind, on the other hand, typically occurs when a person has experienced an upsetting situation or comes into contact with a triggering situation. When people act on their emotions, they tend not to make good choices.

Example: Aaron went on a few dates with a woman to whom he was very attracted. However, when Aaron wanted to take the relationship to the "next step," he knew he had to disclose his sex offender status with the woman. Once he told her that he had been convicted of a sexual offense and was a registered sex offender, the woman became upset, told him that he was "disgusting" and said not to call her ever again.

Staying Safe: My Relapse Prevention Plan

For the final session, begin by asking participants to share which points stood out to them most during treatment and why. Next, spend the first 30–45 minutes reviewing the material from the course.

We learned about the stages of change and that right before someone relapses, they "lapse."[2] The term "lapse" refers to a person reverting back to their immediate triggers, such as viewing excessive pornography, violating terms of probation/parole, having numerous "hook-ups," or masturbating to fantasies about illegal situations.

It is important to have a solid understanding of potentially risky sexual behaviors—including flirting. For the rest of this group, you will begin working on your personal relapse prevention plan. This plan should include only the skills you plan to actually use. Do not include any skills that you are not willing to use. This plan should guide your behaviors when you encounter risky situations. Consider the skills you have learned, practiced, or commit to practicing, and create a sexual safety plan for the future.

Participants may work together to present each other with potentially risky encounters, or responses they may not have considered. The skills trainers will walk around the room and provide participants with feedback. Participants should complete their relapse prevention plan as homework if they do not finish it during group. Once they have completed their relapse prevention plan, they will review it with their individual therapist.

Handout 18.1: My Relapse Prevention Plan

Make sure to keep your relapse prevention plan in an easy-to-locate place.

Coping skills

These are the specific coping skills I will use daily/weekly. Be sure to explain what these will *look* like.

Feeling or situation	Skill(s)

My social supports

Person	Phone number

My Plan of Action for Living a Wise Life

The purpose of the plan of action is to effectively address risky events/ experiences, thoughts, emotions, and behavior. The plan of action should list steps you will take to avoid risky situations for you when they arise.

Situation I will/may encounter	What I will do

Situation I will/may encounter	What I will *not* do

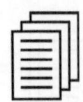

Scheduling my time

Retirement, unemployment, recent release from prison, and too much free time can lead to frequent fantasizing, masturbating, and/or engaging in risky behaviors. Some people find it helpful to schedule their days—including their downtime—in order to ensure they always have something to do and do not get stuck in the trap of feeling bored. You can create a schedule with 15, 30, or 60-minute timeslots—or longer. Be sure to only include activities that you know you will do. Examples may include watching TV, reading a book, meditating, taking a walk, talking to a friend or family member on the phone, etc. Complete a schedule for each day of the week.

Example

Day: Monday

8:00–8:30 am	Eat breakfast and read the news
8.30–9:30 am	Work on my homework
9:30–9:45 am	Practice breathing exercises

My Daily Schedule

Day: _____

Time	Scheduled activity

Notes

1 Wise & Jordan (2021).
2 Ward & Purvis, & Devilly (2004).

References

Ward T., Purvis M., & Devilly G. (2004). Relapse prevention with sex offenders. In McIvor G. and Kemshall H. (eds.), *Research Highlights in Social Work—Sex Offenders: Managing the Risk*. San Francisco, CA: Jessica Kingsley

Wise R.A., & Jordan C.J. (2021). Dopamine, behavior, and addiction. *Journal of Biomedical Science, 28*, 1–9. https://doi.org/10.1186/s12929-021-00779-7

Index